ONE HUNDRED
OF HEALTH

The Changing Health of Guernsey
1899-1999

*Sister, A "first edition,"
— Signed by the editor too .... wow
C.T. isn't the only one to write books

All brotherly love —*

Edited by
Dr David Jeffs
Director of Public Health, States of Guernsey

Guernsey Board of Health
John Henry House
St Martin's, GY4 6UU

First published November 1999

© *All rights reserved. The copyright of individual chapters remains with the contributing authors. No part of this publication may be reproduced or transmitted in any form or by any means including photocopying and recording without written permission of the copyright holder, application for which should be addressed to the Board of Health John Henry House, St Martin's, Guernsey GY4 6UU*

Published by The Board of Health
States of Guernsey
Department of Health, St Martins
Guernsey, Channel Islands, GY4 6UU

First published November 1999

ISBN 1 8999 05 01 4

Printed and bound by
Melody Press Group
L'Islet, Guernsey, CI GY2 4SD

One Hundred Years of Health

Content Summary

Prologue *Setting the Scene* p1

Guernsey in 1900 was far from the healthy semi-rural idyll that we might imagine. Beneath its somewhat bucolic surface lay a very different world where infant mortality was high, deaths from infectious disease were common, and life expectancy was shorter than that of rural Dorset with which the Channel Islands were sometimes compared.

Chapter One *' Through the eyes of the MoH'* p5

In his Annual Report, the Medical Officer of Health (MoH) was required 'to report to his Authority on any influences which were acting in a deleterious manner on the health of the community which he served'. The MoH was also perhaps better placed to view the changing patterns of health and disease in Guernsey than medical colleagues who only saw individual patients. A number of inter-related themes seen 'through the eyes of the MoH' show how the public health of Guernsey has improved over the past one hundred years.

Chapter Two *From Sanitary Reform to Planetary Protection* p23

At the turn of the century, responsibility for sanitation and refuse disposal was firmly vested in the Douzaines and their Parish Constables - powers they were reluctant to surrender. It took 36 years to achieve a uniform approach to environmental health throughout the island, and a further 30 years before the legal **armamentarium** necessary to ensure environmental safety was reasonably complete. In the final one third of the century, environmental concerns have of necessity become more global.

Chapter Three *The story of the Town Hospital* p31

When the Board of Health first met in 1900, the Town Hospital had already existed for over 150years. Although it was to remain independent of the Board until 1970, it never quite lived down the stigma of its origins, having once been a poorhouse. Its few remaining patients were finally transferred to other accommodation in October 1986.

Chapter Four *The Victoria Cottage Hospital (Amherst)* p47

The 'respectable poor' were reluctant to seek admission to either the Town or Country Hospitals because of the perceived stigma of their 'Poor Law' origins. Dr E Laurie Robinson had the vision to propose a "Guernsey Cottage Hospital," and the drive and determination to seek the funds needed to turn this vision into reality. The Victoria Hospital was in turn Cottage Hospital, hospital for British Troops during World War One, for German Troops during World War Two, and finally a maternity home before the last patients left in March 1980.

Chapter Five *Mental Health Services* p57

The care of the mentally unwell was long linked with the care of other indigents. Although the need for improved provision of care was identified in the 1930s, it was not until after World War Two that a specialist psychiatric service began to develop. The Castel Hospital was central to the care of the mentally ill throughout this period, until the concepts of 'community care' began to be accepted in the 1970s.

Chapter Six *Looking after Learning Disabilities* p63

In 1930, it was reported that 'such a competent body as the Mental Deficiency Committee estimates that the proportion of population mentally sub-normal (in Guernsey) is no less than 10%." This personal account captures what it was like to care for children with learning disabilities in the 1960s and ends optimistically with plans and hopes for the future.

Chapter Seven *Health services for children* p69

Concern about the poor physical state of many army recruits led to the establishment of the School Medical Services in Britain in the early years of this century. Other nations, notably the United States and Germany followed. Despite repeated calls for a School Medical Service in Guernsey, the first School Nurses were only appointed in 1927, and it was a further ten years before a part-time School's Medical Officer was appointed. During the post war years, the Service has developed in complexity and range, to meet the changing health needs of different generations of students.

Chapter Eight *The Community Nursing Services* p79

For the great part of this century, most births, and deaths and much medical care took place outside hospital, in people's homes and other community settings. Essential to the delivery of this care were the nurses of the three Guernsey District Nursing Associations. The contribution of community nurses, and the increasing specialisation of their roles forms the theme of this chapter.

Chapter Nine *Health in the Occupation* p87

Bereft by evacuation of most of its younger people, in June 1940 the population of Guernsey aged almost overnight. Planning for the War emergency and then the Occupation forced rapid and radical reform of health services. The Occupation saw clear improvements in maternity care, but the most significant contribution to health came from States intervention to maximise food production and ensure fair distribution.

Chapter Ten *The post war period* p99

While the National Health Service was being established in Britain, Guernsey chose to follow a different course. The growth of group practice, with 'generalists' and 'specialists ' working alongside one another became the established pattern. Several local doctors recall experiences in a system which was unusual in Europe, although more common in countries such as Australia and Canada.

Chapter Eleven *Pressures for change - A Specialist View* p111

Technical advances, increasing specialisation, and rising health care together led to tensions within the group practices, and confrontation with States Committees. The medical profession recognised the need for change, but it was political pressure that eventually forced the separation of primary from secondary care, and led to the formation of the Medical Specialist Group. This in turn paved the way for the introduction of the Health Insurance Scheme.

Chapter Twelve *Paying for Health* p121

The increasing complexities of health care led inevitably to escalating costs. Following the separation of secondary care under the Medical Specialist Group, the 1991 Census suggested that a sizeable minority of Guernsey's population might be excluded from seeking necessary specialist care by financial barriers. The changing philosophies of health care funding in Guernsey are explored, and the pressures which led to the development and implementation of the Health Insurance Scheme explained.

Chapter Thirteen *Two Complementary Guernsey Physicians* p135

The facts covering the evolution of health care in Guernsey over the past one hundred years are more easily recounted than depicting the human element which made such changes possible. Here two complementary portraits of two 'complementary Guernsey physicians' are included to illustrate this human dimension.

Chapter Fourteen *The Ambulance and Rescue Service* p143

That Guernsey never developed an ambulance service run by the States was largely due to the vision and drive of one islander - Reginald Blanchford - who founded a unique ambulance and rescue service covering land, sea and air. Under his successors this has developed into a comprehensive modern service, which must be the envy of many other island communities around the world.

Chapter Fifteen *Health care in Alderney* p155

The Board of Health's mandate requires that it 'maintain and improve the health of the people of Guernsey and Alderney'. The history of health in the northern isle has of necessity taken a somewhat different course to the path in Guernsey, but increasingly since the involvement of the Board of Health these separate paths are converging.

Chapter Sixteen *The changing mandate of the Board of the Health* p165

The evolving role and responsibility of the Board is charted by a series of 'snapshots' of important decisions of the States of Guernsey. In particular the Board's responsibility for managing and developing the islands healthcare institutions and its more recent role in commissioning more comprehensive health services to islanders is examined.

Appendix: Presidents of the Board of Health, Medical Officers of Health, Hospital Secretaries/Administrators/Chief Executives

Illustrations and Acknowledgements

p19	Collecting water around 1900	
p20	Public pump in Cornet Street around 1900	*Courtesy* Guerin Collection, Guernsey Press
p21	Collecting milk in Guernsey can	
p22	Sedan Chair in St Peter Port	
	Guernsey grocery shop around 1910	*Courtesy* States Archives
p43	Town Hospital Picnic and Imperial Hotel Pleinmont 1911	*Courtesy* Mrs Gillian Lenfestey
p44	At the Town Hospital Christmas Day 1938	*Courtesy* Carel Toms Collection and Mrs Gillian Lenfestey
p45	The Victoria Cottage Hospital	*Courtesy* Carel Toms Collection and W T (Bill) Gallienne
p46	Valnord House and Floraville	*Courtesy* Mrs Sylvia Hickman
p97/98	Health during the Occupation	*Courtesy* Reg Blanchford and St John Ambulance and Rescue Service
p109/10	Royal Visits 1949 & 1975	*Courtesy* States Board of Health
p119	Surgery at the Country Hospital and the PEH	*Courtesy* Dr Jim Dickson
p119	The Bailiff opens Alexandra House	*Courtesy* Medical Specialist Group
p120	Guernsey's oldest X-ray?	*Courtesy* Dr Jonathan Hanaghan
p153/54	Sea, Air and Land	*Courtesy* St John Ambulance and Rescue Service
p163	Opening of Mignot Hospital	*Courtesy* Mr Brian Bonnard
p163	German orthopaedic instruments	*Courtesy* Alderney Gazette
p164	PEH Hospital - Then and Now	*Courtesy* States Board of Health

Contributor Profiles

Dr David Jeffs

Dr David Jeffs has been Director of Public Health in Guernsey since 1994. He has a particular interest in medical history, having previously published on Naval surgeons and early exploration, and the Plague in Australia 1900-1910.

Mr John Cook

Arriving in Guernsey in 1979, John Cook worked first as an Environmental Health Officer, becoming Deputy Chief Environmental Health Officer in 1986, and is now Chief Environmental Health Officer (designate). He has particular interests in the broader aspects of environmental protection.

Mrs Gillian Lenfestey

Mrs Gillian Lenfestey is married to the first Island Archivist, now retired, was a research assistant for several years, and is Costume Curator to the National Trust of Guernsey. She was co-editor of a 'History of Presbyterianism in Guernsey' and has written a study of medical practices at the Town Hospital in the 18th and 19th centuries.

Mr W T (Bill) Gallienne

W T (Bill) Gallienne is Guernsey born, and spent many years as Assistant Archivist assisting in setting up the Island Archives Service, an account of which he has published. He is the President of La Société Guernesiaise, a Trustee of the Millennium Tapestry Trust, and an active member of Le Cercle Français de Guernesey, the Society of Archivists and of Les Ravigotteurs.

Mr Adrian Gaggs

Adrian Gaggs trained in psychology at Manchester and Leeds Universities before going to work in various psychiatric settings in Switzerland. He has now worked in Guernsey for nineteen years, developing particular research interests in alcohol, addictions, eating disorders, and the elderly.

Mrs Sylvia Hickman

Mrs Sylvia Hickman was born in Guernsey and is secretary of the Archaeological Section of La Société Guernesiaise and chairperson of The Guernsey Writers' Circle. Previous publications include travel articles in the Guernsey Press.

Mr Richard Hocart

Richard Hocart is Administration Manager at the office of the States Education Council. His published historical work includes a study of the development of the States of Guernsey and a biography of Sir Peter de Havilland.

Mrs Ann Jones

Anne Jones has a background in community nursing and midwifery and has worked in clinical practice in Newfoundland Canada, and in various posts in the North West of England. She came to Guernsey in 1998 as a Community Tutor based at the Nurse Education Centre.

Mr Ken Tough

Ken Tough was born in Guernsey in 1948. He read history at Cambridge and returned to Guernsey in 1970 to join the Civil Service. In 1981 he was appointed H.M. Greffier. He has been Review Editor of the Channel Islands Occupation Society (Guernsey) since 1993.

Dr Brian Seth-Smith

Brian Seth-Smith came to Guernsey in 1960 as a general surgeon, obtaining a partnership in one of the six group practices. As was the established custom then, he took part in general practice for several years. He later served as medical member of the Board of Health and Chairman of the PEH Medical Staff Committee. He took part in the early planning of the Medical Specialist Group (MSG).

Mr Roger Allsopp

A 1964 Durham graduate, Roger Allsopp obtained his FRCS in 1970 and completed his higher surgical training in 1975, when he joined the Grange End Practice as a partner. He then obtained a Master's Degree in Medical Law from Cardiff University in 1990. He was closely involved in the formation of the MSG and the negotiations leading to the Specialist Health Insurance Scheme and the Specialist Contract.

Dr Stephen Langford

Dr Stephen Langford is the Chief Executive Officer of the States Housing Authority. He was formerly the Administration Director at the Board of Health and the Deputy Chief Executive of the Guernsey Social Security Authority. He was a member of the team of officers which negotiated the Specialist Health Insurance Scheme contracts with the Medical Specialist Group and Ophthalmic Group, and has played a prominent role in the review of the funding of long-term care services.

Rev L G H Craske

After war service in the Hussars, the Rev Leslie Craske graduated at King's College University of London, where he was elected as President of the University Union. He is a Scholar in Theology in Latin studies. After years as a missionary priest in Africa, he returned to London to be vicar of Upper Norwood. He now lives in St Peter Port.

Mr Neil Tucker

After leaving University with a degree in physics, Neil Tucker began work for a large bank in the UK. He spent all his spare time with the St John Ambulance organisation, and pursued this vocation when he moved to Guernsey, where he was recruited by Reg. Blanchford into the professional St John Ambulance & Rescue Service. He became a principal member of the cliff rescue team, an operator of the mobile radar unit, and qualified as an ambulance service instructor. He was the Service's training officer before becoming Chief Ambulance Officer in 1990.

Mr Philip Cranford-Smith

Mr Philip Cranford-Smith has lived in Alderney since 1980 where he has worked both as schools dentist and in private practice. Now retired, he has taken a keen interest in Alderney politics, where he is the Member of the States of Alderney with special responsibility for health matters, and is also a representative of Alderney in the States of Guernsey.

Mr Alan Hodgkinson

Mr Alan Hodgkinson has been Chief Executive of the Board of Health since March 1992. He trained and qualified as a health care administrator in the NHS before moving to the private sector where he spent ten years working for BUPA hospitals. He is particularly interested in healthcare systems, their origins and effectiveness.

Special Acknowledgements:

Special thanks are due to local historian Dr Gregory Stevens Cox who has acted as mentor to the project, made his own contribution, and offered several other useful suggestions.

A special thanks too to Mrs Yvonne Kaill who has been invaluable in transcribing the various contributions, liaising with printers, and ensuring the project met its several deadlines: Dr David Jeffs [Editor]

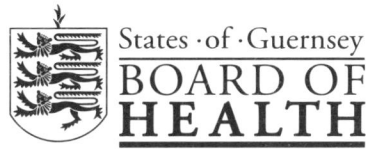

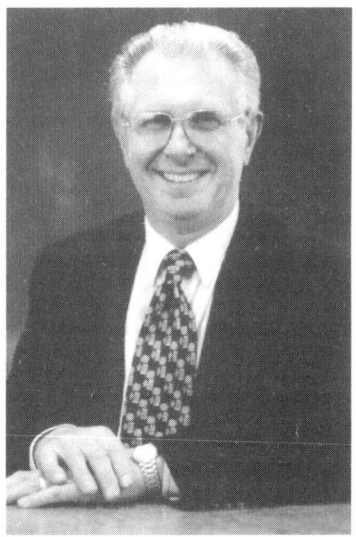

FOREWORD

To those of us who are around the age when we could draw a pension, one hundred years may not seem such a long time.

But the fact that we are here at all, and that most of us enjoy reasonably good health underscores the huge and amazing improvements in health that have been achieved in Guernsey during the past one hundred years.

It is very easy to forget that at the beginning of the century, only about one quarter of the population reached the aged of 65 or above, and there were times when almost one child in four died before their first birthday.

Even in the middle years of this century, many of us can remember, when there were outbreaks of diphtheria and polio, and islanders spent months at a time in 'the Sanatorium' waiting for their tuberculous lungs to heal sufficiently so that they no longer posed a health threat to the wider community.

This must seem like another world to young people growing up in Guernsey today, and I feel this timely publication of *'One Hundred Years of Health'* will therefore appeal to all ages, the older ones of us who remember many of the incidents and personalities described, whilst the younger generation will be fascinated by how much life and health has changed since their parents and their grandparents were young.

Such improvements and health have not been achieved by one group alone. The medical profession has made important contributions, but so too have nurses in our hospitals and in the community, our unique local St John Ambulance and Rescue, and the many ordinary men and women of our island, who have given their time to serve on committees, to raise funds for charitable institutions, and to care for their own sick loved ones outside our hospitals. To all of them we owe a debt of gratitude for the much improved health we enjoy today.

But as these pages show, much of this would not have happened, or would have happened in a very different way without the existence and involvement of the States Board of Health. As the Board celebrates 'One Hundred Years of Health' and prepares to enter its second century and the new Millennium, I feel proud to have been elected President, and on behalf of my Board, proud of what has been achieved.

My congratulations to the editor and contributors of this publication for bringing this fascinating story to us. I commend it to you, I hope you enjoy and learn from it.

Deputy Brian Russell
President, States Board of Health

Prologue

Dr David Jeffs

Guernsey in 1900 was far from the healthy semi-rural idyll that we might imagine. Beneath its somewhat bucolic surface lay a very different world where infant mortality was high, deaths from infectious disease were common, and life expectancy was shorter than that of rural Dorset with which the Channel Islands were sometimes compared.

Setting the scene ....

The summers of the late 1890's in Guernsey were generally fine ones, with average summer temperatures around two degrees warmer than those recorded in the previous decade.

As the century neared its end, the British Empire, of which Guernsey was a proud part, basked in the golden glow of late imperial splendour.

Two years previously, on 22nd June 1897, her Majesty Queen Victoria had celebrated her Diamond Jubilee by being driven in an open carriage from Buckingham Palace down Pall Mall, the Strand and Fleet Street to a special commemorative service in front of St Paul's Cathedral. She was accompanied by representatives of most of the crowned heads of Europe, Crown Princes and Grand Dukes, Indian Princes and Oriental Potentates, Governors from the Colonies and Foreign Ambassadors.

The day was bright and sunny with white fluffy clouds, - *'Queen's weather'* the people called it. As well as contingents from the leading Regiments of the British Army, there were representatives from all over the Empire, Australian Cavalry, Indian Lancers, marching troops and bands, each in their own distinctive uniforms. Included too was a contingent from the Royal Guernsey Militia - in all around 50,000 troops forming part of the *'the largest military force ever assembled in London'*.

The procession was watched by a huge crowd, subdued at first, then progressively more jubilant in their acclaim as the procession gathered way.

A special supplement to the Guernsey Evening Star reported on Tuesday 24th June 1897, *'There may have been 250,000, there may have been half a million, there may have been more. Never was a greater multitude within these limits ..... all the people of the world seemed to be gathered for this grand pageant.'*

Most people at the time, whether observers of the procession itself, or later reading the glowing accounts of the occasion in their newspapers, must have mused no doubt, that this was indeed the British Empire at its zenith.

As the century moved to its conclusion however, a different mood seemed to take hold. In closeby France, a certain weariness or *ennui,* a reaction perhaps against the perceived decadence of the 'naughty Nineties' seemed to take over.

The French described it as *'fin de siecle'* a feeling that one age was coming to an end, and a new era was about to begin.

In Britain too, the mood was more sombre and subdued. What had seemed in September 1899 as merely continuing colonial problems in faraway South Africa, had by December of that year escalated into open conflict with the Boer farmers of the Transvaal and Orange Free State. Far from being the latest in the series of small colonial wars which had engaged the British Army almost continuously since Waterloo, they found themselves fighting perhaps their first modern war. Embarking with confidence, they had suffered early and unexpected military reverses on several fronts.

Guernsey in 1899

With its large French speaking population, the small but loyal Crown Dependency of Guernsey - then an island of around 40,000 population seemed to catch the prevailing moods of both France and Britain.

The wreck of the *'Stella'* on the Casquets off Alderney, with the loss of over 100 lives in March of that year had dealt a serious blow to the developing tourist industry. Prices for horticultural produce had been low, whilst the local press grimly reported the *'very heavy losses'* and *'a terrible list of casualties'* in successive engagements in the South African War.

The weather too had turned unseasonably cold. The Guernsey Star reported on the 14th December 1899, '*A fall of snow heavier than any known for several years, followed by a severe frost with many exposed sheets of water frozen'*.

The newly published Guernsey Evening Press perhaps best summarised the mood of the Islands in its New Year's Editorial to it readers dated Monday 1st January 1900.

'1899 and another year has slipped away, a year full of stirring events in the world at large, and our island home also. In neither case, unfortunately, can we say all has been for the best .... the present war entered upon with a light heart against two insignificant and supposed half civilised Republics, has shown how the conditions of warfare have altered, the flower of our troops and the pick of our officers have suffered defeats such as England has not been accustomed to.

Here at home, the dreadful disaster of the Stella at the very commencement of our real business year, was an awful start to our tourist season. It is certain that most tradesmen in the island have not had a busy time, the year has not been a good one as far as trade is concerned .... nothing has been done to improve financial conditions of the island ...... there is every prospect of a serious deficit or greatly enhanced taxation. That a general re-organisation of States finances must soon come about is evident, for with the Railway Companies on one side clamouring for reduced harbour fees, and growers on the other requiring relief from wharfage charges, and an incessant expenditure, it is evident the old system cannot stand much longer'.

It was against this background that the States met at the end of December 1899 to deliberate *'whether they are of the opinion to appoint a Consultative Committee to look after the public health ....'*. This matter was not as straightforward as might be supposed, and was hotly debated. It was only after the intervention of Her Majesty's Procuerer did the States vote in favour.

Here at least was some small cause for celebration. The Editor of the Guernsey Evening Press commented *'Public health also has been unsatisfactory .... but some good is being done in as much as the Authorities have now been aroused and better preventative measures will be taken in the future........'*

The nine members of the first States Board of Health duly met under the chairmanship of General H le Cocq some one week later. Guernsey's first Medical Officer of Health, Dr John Brownlea MD, DPH, who had taken up his appointment some months previously, was in attendance.

'One Hundred Years of Health'

What brought these nine prominent citizens together, *'the better preventative measures'* which have since been implemented and some of the people and events which have helped shape health in Guernsey in the one hundred years since then are the theme of this book.

It would be impossible to do justice to such a broad subject in a single volume. Instead, we present a series of perspectives on different topics, and by a number of authors.

These are arranged roughly in chronological order, but inevitably there is some overlap, and the need for a certain amount of cross-referencing. However, taken together they do go some way to illuminating the huge improvements in the health of our island during this period, and how this has been accomplished.

For huge improvements in health there undoubtedly have been. The Guernsey pictured in the prints of the Guerin Collection, a number of which are included in this volume, depict a Guernsey which in its essentials is easily recognisable today.

The majority of the Guerin prints date *'from the three or four hectic years before 1900'* - the period when the events which were ultimately to lead to the formation of the Board of Health were beginning to unfold.

Looking at these strangely familiar scenes of streets devoid of motor vehicles, of fresh produce piled high on market stalls, of unhurried citizens in both town and country enjoying a seemingly tranquil pace of life, it is easy to imagine that the population of this semi-rural idyll, with its bracing and invigorating maritime climate, must have enjoyed excellent health. Guernsey itself appears to have believed so.

Unfortunately however, the facts tell a somewhat different story. In 1900 the average age of death in Guernsey was under 40 years, lower than rural Dorset with which the Channel Islands were sometimes compared. One hundred years later, life expectancy is now closer to 80 years.

Then little over one person in four would reach the age of 65 years, whilst today 80% of all male deaths and 87% of all female deaths in Guernsey occur in people above this age, and it is likely that these trends will continue.

In 1900, around one quarter all children born in the Parish of St Sampsons died before celebrating their first birthday. The infant mortality rate in St Sampsons was described as *'being higher than that of the poorest, most densely populated part of Liverpool ......'*. Today less than five children in every thousand born in Guernsey die before their first year of life, a decline in infant mortality of over 97% in just one hundred years.

It is axiomatic to historical research that *'to comprehend the present, we must first understand the past'*. If you are interested in the social history of Guernsey, in the changing patterns of health and disease on the island, in why we have the health system which has evolved, why this is different from almost anywhere else in Europe, and how this has been achieved, then here is a story for you. This is how it began.......................

Chapter One

' Through the eyes of the MoH '

Dr David Jeffs

In his Annual Report, the Medical Officer of Health (MoH) was required 'to report to his Authority on any influences which were acting in a deleterious manner on the health of the community which he served'. The MoH was also perhaps better placed to view the changing patterns of health and disease in Guernsey than medical colleagues who only saw individual patients. A number of inter-related themes seen 'through the eyes of the MoH' show how the public health of Guernsey has improved over the past one hundred years .

How it began......

When I took up my appointment as Guernsey's ninth Medical Officer of Health (MoH) in the spring of 1994, an early call was to inspect a collection of large cardboard boxes which had apparently been gathering dust for several years in the basement of Lukis House in the Grange, St Peter Port. Inside I found old glass syringes with needles that could be resharpened and reused - no doubt a remnant of the TB clinic? There were also strange wooden boxes containing antiquated electrical equipment which I imagined must once have been used in the treatment of venereal disease? There were dusty pamphlets from the Ministry of Health advising on the management of polio and the prevention of rickets and other now largely forgotten diseases. But I also found one box containing some twenty or so volumes of bound Reports, the early ones with worn leather bindings and faded gold titles, the more recent volumes being merely bound with cloth covers. These were the Annual Reports of the Medical Officer of Health for Guernsey.

In fairly short time, I found myself needing to report *'on the health of the island '* for my own Annual Reports, and I sometimes found myself flicking through these old volumes, interested to see how my predecessors had viewed a particular problem.

As I read their various accounts and reports, so I began to appreciate the personalities of the individual writers. Some I could quickly warm to as old friends, others never became more than shadowy figures from the past. However, as I studied their various narratives, I began to reflect on how much health in Guernsey had changed over the past one hundred years, yet how much the problems had remained the same. Here I thought, was a story worth re-telling.

But how to translate this mass of information into a form which could be read, understood and enjoyed by the general reader? As I considered further, it struck me that there were a number of inter-related themes which together told the story far better than any mere chronological sequence. So why not let the men who had experienced these events first hand, the qualified physicians who were perhaps best placed to appreciate the importance of the events they described re-tell these in their own words? Here then are some aspects of changing health in Guernsey *'through the eyes of the MoH'*.

An outbreak of diphtheria

Diphtheria is a disease of the upper respiratory tract caused by the organism *'Corynebacterium diphtheriae'* It has a 2-5 day incubation period with fever and the development of a characteristic adherent greyish membrane of the throat said to be caused by a cytoxin. In the more severe cases, there may be gross swelling of the neck which can lead to respiratory obstruction and death.

Before the late 1880's diphtheria had been relatively rare on Guernsey. Then between 1887 and 1893, there had been 38 deaths from diphtheria, croup and laryngitis (grouped together because of uncertainties of diagnosis). This averaged a rate of 6 per year. By 1895, deaths from these causes had increased to 20 per year, and as a consequence diphtheria was made a notifiable disease in that year. Between 1895 and 1898, 62 deaths were recorded from diphtheria, an increase to over 20 deaths per year.

The summers of the 1890's are remembered for being particularly long and dry, and some blamed the weather for the steady increase in cases *'1899 was a dry year ...... one of a series in which there has been deficient rainfall, and as often happens with such periods of prolonged relative drought, diphtheria has advanced both in extent and severity'*.

In 1899 there were in fact to be 121 cases of diphtheria and 23 deaths. However, these were not evenly distributed, with 43 cases of diphtheria, but only one death in the Town (a mortality rate of 2.3%), compared with 78 cases and 22 deaths in the country (a mortality rate over twelve times as great at almost 30%).

Action was obviously necessary, and the Royal Court therefore appointed a Committee *'for the purpose of considering the measures necessary to combat the disease'* (diphtheria). On 29th March 1899, the Report of the Committee was accepted by the States.

The Committee reported that *'the main causes of the outbreaks of diphtheria, scarlet fever and enteric fever was the unsanitary state of certain houses and localities due to defective drainage, cesspools, accumulations of household refuse, manure heaps and pits, pig sties, and latrines, etc in close proximity to drinking water. making it a source of constant danger.*

They recommended that a Medical Officer of Health be appointed at a salary of £200 per year and *'with the powers necessary to combat the illnesses'*. In April it was further agreed that *'a laboratory was to be fitted out at the expense of about £100'*, whilst in May the Castel Hospital Authorities agreed to lend the isolation hospital for a period of six months in an attempt to control the epidemic.

However these measures by themselves were not sufficient, and in July the States agreed to accept responsibility for the expense of admission and isolation. In the autumn of 1899, a series of six lectures relating to public health were arranged by the Royal Court and given at the Guilles Alles Meeting Rooms, whilst in October Guernsey's first Medical Officer of Health Dr John Brownlea MD DPH arrived on the Island.

Appointment of the Board of Health

In its Report accepted by the States in March 1899, the Committee of the Royal Court had stated, *'that present laws give ample power to Parochial Authorities, but laws are useless unless applied and observed'*. They added *'dangers to public health still exist'* and suggested *'that a central Board of Health be appointed'*.

In due course, at the States meeting on 29th December 1899 the States were asked to deliberate *'whether they are of the opinion to appoint a Consulting Committee to look after the public health, to advise and co-operate with the Parochial Sanitary Committees of the Island with a view to ensuring effective general application of all measures necessary to safeguard the public health, and to propose such modifications or additions to the laws and ordinances that may be thought necessary'*.

Powers for regulating sanitation and refuse disposal had been given to the Parish Authorities in St Peter Port in 1853, and extended to the Douzaines and Constables in the Country Parishes in 1865. It had been described as *'a very comprehensive law ... which may have been in advance of any legislation of the kind elsewhere'*.

The Douzaines were understandably not willing to give up such powers easily. At the States Debate on 29th December, the Deputy for St Peter in the Woods stated *'At present the Douzaines were the only Sanitation Committees in the Parishes. It was now suggested that they should be subservient to a States Committee. They could not accept this position He proposed an amendment that the Douzaines continued to be the only Committees in their respective Parishes, that the services of the Health Officer remain at the disposal of the Parishes, and that the Constables of the Parishes report on sanitary conditions of their Parishes at each Chief Pleas'*. The Deputy for the Castel seconded the amendment and there appeared to be wide general support for this view within the States.

However, Deputy Collenette of the Town Parish countered *'He had paid a great deal of attention to sanitation. Our death rate had risen in the past 30 years, and it had not been prevented by the ancient system, because that system had broken down'*.

'Do the Parochial Authorities possess the knowledge required?' he asked, *'Can we expect visitors or commercial success without a clean bill of health and a low death rate? Mistakes were constantly being made by the Parochial Authorities - the cost entailed* (in the new arrangements) *would be more than met by the increased prosperity of the Island'*.

The matter still hung in the balance when Her Majesty's Procureur made some conciliatory remarks *'He thought the Constables and Douzaineers were trying to do their duty and were waking up to the threatening position. However, if we do not put our affairs in order from a sanitary point of view, then we may get some epidemic'*.

'He could not understand why some looked upon a Committee of the States with suspicion. It was only intended to form a consultative committee to lay down such principles of health as were adopted all over the world. The Douzaines were not to be deprived of their power, but were to be helped......'.

The Procureur's view seems to have swung the argument, and it was agreed to appoint a Committee of *'nine members elected by the States, the three oldest members retiring each year, but eligible for re-election. The Senior Jurat of the Committee to be President, and the Supervisor to be an ex-officio member'*. One week later on Saturday 6th January 1900, the newly appointed Board of Health met for the first time. General H le Cocq was Chairman, other members were Jurat Ozanne, the Reverend H W Brock, and Messrs Valpied, Collenette, J W Dorey, Collas and Foote.

At its first meeting, the Board agreed '*A statement of all infectious cases and the comments from the MoH thereon shall be read and discussed at each meeting'*, but *'that all professional matters should be left to the MoH, except where he wishes advice'*.

Diphtheria outbreak controlled

On the advice of the Medical Officer of Health, public health measures were soon instituted, including the equipment of a laboratory, the isolation of infectious cases in the 'Country Hospital' at States expense whenever necessary, and the limited use of the new 'diphtheria antitoxin'. These new measures were soon to prove effective, and from 120 cases and 23 deaths from diphtheria in 1899, there were 80 cases and 34 deaths in 1900, 66 cases and 19 deaths in 1901, and 179 cases but only 16 deaths in 1902.

In 1903 the King Edward Sanatorium was opened at a cost of £6,500. 113 patients were admitted in the first year, of whom 83 had diphtheria. There were 9 deaths. By 1904, the worst was clearly over - 55 cases of diphtheria, but only one death. Guernsey's third Medical Officer of Health, Dr Henry Draper Bishop was able to comment *'I am of the opinion that but for the efficient machinery that is now in operation for checking the disease, serious epidemic extensions would have occurred'*.

The developing role of the MoH

The Committee of the Royal Court had initially recommended that a Medical Officer of Health should be appointed for only three years - perhaps the authorities hoped that once diphtheria was under control, that the position could be dispensed with? In the event Dr John Brownlea was to stay for little over one year, before departing to take up the new position of Physician Superintendent at the Glasgow Fever Hospital.

He was replaced by Dr E Stanley Hoare who left abruptly in September 1902 following a disagreement with the Board of Health over additional payments for looking after patients at the newly completed King Edward Sanatorium.

Guernsey's third Medical Officer of Health in as many years was Dr Henry Draper Bishop who took up office in 1903, and was to become the longest serving Medical Officer, eventually retiring in 1934 at the age of 70.

But with diphtheria now apparently under control, what should be the role of the newly appointed Medical Officer of Health? Dr Henry Draper Bishop wrote in 1904;

'With the many natural advantages we enjoy in this highly favoured island, and the absence of factories and injurious trades, coupled with the large area that might be described as 'rural' I cannot help thinking that our death rate should be lower than it has been in the past......' He set out to tackle these other causes of poor health and premature death, and in doing so, established the foundations on which our present system of public health is built.

Dr Bishop remarked one year later, *'It is the duty of the MoH to be an enthusiast, perhaps even a dreamer. The Board whose servant he will decide whether his suggestions are practical or not.'* And during the 32 years he was to hold the position of MoH, Dr Bishop commented tirelessly on his concerns - factors which he felt could adversely affect the health of the population.

Amongst these factors were the growth in population, inadequate housing standards, concerns about food and water quality, the need for better sewerage and sanitation, waste disposal, hospital efficiency, and the need for better public health information. Many of his concerns sound remarkably familiar to the modern ear.

The need for health information

Epidemiology or the collection and analysis of health statistics forms the basis of modern public health. When Dr John Brownlea had arrived in Guernsey in 1899, he was horrified to find there was no system of registration of cause of death. *'The system regarding these is so imperfect that they can only be used as rough indications and not as trustworthy guides'* he wrote.

The same theme was continued by Dr E Stanley Hoare the following year *'the records I found at the Health Office were rather meagre'*, whilst Dr Henry Draper Bishop was rather more forceful, writing in 1902;

'The system of death registration obtaining in Guernsey is very unsatisfactory as a large number of deaths are registered without any medical certificate of death being produced. Apart from the very obvious dangers of such a system, it is difficult to get satisfactory statistics when such a comprehensive but vague statement as "complications of disease" is given as a cause of death.

'My predecessors have called attention to the urgent necessity of a revision of the law dealing with this matter, and an admirable "Projet de Loi" has been prepared (by the Board of Health) *and submitted to the Crown Law Officers, which I honestly hope the Royal Court will soon see fit to pass'.*

However, the Crown Law Officers obviously did not share this sense of urgency, and it was not until 1909 that the *'Registration of Cause of Death'* Law was finally implemented, after over six years delay.

Deficiencies in health data in other fields were also apparent, and were slowly rectified but usually only after a struggle. *'The Registration of Stillbirths'* became law in Guernsey from 1st April 1907, but the routine notification of births did not become compulsory until nine years later.

Henry Draper Bishop pointed out the value of this measure in *'assisting directly in the reduction of infantile mortality. It directs that the father or other persons stated shall notify the MoH within 36 hours of the birth of a child. In the poorer districts, the mother is visited by a Health Visitor - a trained nurse, who advises the mother as to the bringing up of the child'*. However, it was to be 1915 before the *'Early Notification of Births'* Act was passed by the Royal Court, and 1946 before the first two Health Visitors were appointed in Guernsey.

Moreover, the deaths of mothers during childbirth were still not being notified in the 1930's and it was only the crisis of 1933, with nine maternal deaths being recorded in a single year that finally forced action in this regard as is described below.

Reliable and timely health information remains the key to improving health, and even in the 1990's Guernsey's health information systems, although improving, remain deficient in many respects.

Other public health concerns

The rambling streets of St Peter Port and St Sampsons may seem picturesque enough today, but at the turn of the century they frequently hid overcrowded, insanitary and unhealthy living conditions. The need for improvements in living conditions were to be a continuing theme of Dr Henry Draper Bishop's Reports.

With regard to housing standards he commented *'There can be no doubt that overcrowding exists in parts of the Island and that highly congested districts are to be met with especially in the urban areas .... The number of persons thus herded together is often so great that health, cleanliness and morality cannot but suffer under these conditions.'* [MoH Report 1903]

'No one expects anything but weeds to grow on rubbish heaps, or flowers to flourish unless care be taken with the soil in which they grow; neither can we expect healthy bodies and minds if people are herded together under impossible conditions.' [MoH Report 1908]

And later *'It is the duty of an MoH to consider the housing question as one of the most important questions with which he is concerned, and on looking over my past Reports, I find I devoted a great deal of space year after year to this question.'* [MoH Report 1921]

'Up to the present time not a single house erected by the States contains a bathroom, ... if only the inhabitants of Guernsey were as well provided for in the matter of baths as they were with churches and chapels, then there would be no cause for complaint'. [MoH Report 1927]

He also identified food and water as important prerequisites for maintaining the public health. He wrote;
'Adulteration of foods chiefly affects the poorer classes and should be kept in check as much as possible by constant and vigorous action on the part of the Authorities, so that it will not pay people to sell adulterated food on account of the risk of detection. [MoH Report 1913]

With regard to water quality he wrote *'Good health is impossible when contaminated water is habitually taken, no very definite sickness may result from it as a certain amount of immunity from continued use may develop, but anaemia, sore throats, loss of appetite, digestive and intestinal disturbances are some of the symptoms of the chronic poisoning which are usually present.'* [MoH Report 1911]

The fight for legislation

It was obvious that in order to tackle problems as diverse as poor housing, sanitation, food and water quality, that better public health legislation was required. Public health in England had been regulated by the 'great' *Public Health Act* of 1875, which dealt in a comprehensive way with such matters as nuisances, offensive trades, unsound food, infectious diseases, the prevention of epidemics, the regulation of markets and slaughter houses, and the making of local government bylaws.

However, it will be recalled that in Guernsey, the States had voted that the Board of Health should be an advisory committee only, and that existing statutory powers should remain with the Parish Constables. The history of progress in public health in Guernsey over the next thirty five years is largely the story of repeated attempts to give Guernsey the same level of statutory protection that England had enjoyed since 1875. No one felt these deficiencies more keenly than Henry Draper Bishop.

'When one comes to the remedying of sanitary defects', he wrote *'it is another matter, so many different authorities have to be consulted, and these authorities are so frequently changed that it is often difficult to get these matters attended to, the process is both indirect and cumbersome, and the source of much extra work to the Board and its officials. The want of this law which should have preceded the recent drainage works has prevented our having definite requirements as regards sanitary matters'.* [MoH Report 1902]

And again *'Sanitary administration continues in great measure to be still carried out by the Douzaines. I think the time is now arrived when the Board of Health should be invested with more powers and responsibilities.'* [MoH Report 1908]

These deficiencies were also supported by some States members, and a Requete was proposed in the Billet d'Etat of 11th December 1912 in which;

'The Petitioners state that it is their conviction that the existing system, whereby the Douzaine of each Parish is its sanitary authority and the Board of Health an advisory committee only, had in practice proved a failure, the island was in their opinion, too small for ten executive bodies and one consultative body to exercise their functions with advantage to the community.'

On account of pressure of business, the Requete was not considered by the States until early in 1913, when the States agreed to establish a Committee of Enquiry.

This Committee duly reported (Billet d'Etat 29th April 1914) suggesting that *'the powers given to the States Sanitary Committee were amply sufficient to safeguard the health of the island if full use were made of its powers.'*

With this recommendation, the States decided to take no further action, and the lack of statutory authority accorded to the Board of Health remained unchanged. It seems that this decision reflected the views of many islanders, for it was reported *'with regards to one effective Sanitary Authority the majority of people in Guernsey are either apathetic or hostile to the creation of such.'*

Dr Henry Draper Bishop appears to have accepted this reverse stoically, writing;

'No doubt the Board would prefer to have a larger share of responsibility, and so would its Medical Officer of Health. There are many who blame the Board of Health for the existing state of things, but when the Board on many occasions has sought increased powers, the States have not granted them, and it is evident that the majority of the people prefer things as they are.' [MoH Report 1919]

However, he did not give up, writing some years later; *'It is very difficult for the MoH to produce satisfactory reports year by year, as amongst the various Authorities concerned with the public health are the ten Parish Douzaines and their Constables, the Board of Health, the Board of Administration, the Island Drainage Board, the Construction of Houses Committee and the Island Sanitation Committee. Some of these Authorities issue reports and some do not, so the MoH is not cognisant in many cases of the work which they have accomplished'* [MoH Report 1931]

Eventually his persistence and perseverance paid off and in 1932, the States finally agreed to increased powers for the Board of Health. However, the proposed *'Loi Relative a la Santé Publique'* only paralleled the 1875 Public Health Act in England, and was not enacted until 1934. It was 1936 before the supporting Ordinance was passed.

Dr Henry Draper Bishop commented *'The difficulties of dual control and of having eleven Sanitary Authorities in such a small Island were apparent to the Board, and it was felt that this was only possible solution of the present impasse'*.

Tackling infant mortality

The granting of new powers to the Board of Health did not however tackle all public health concerns - the high infant mortality rate being one such. Dr Henry Draper Bishop had written in 1904 *'The infantile death of St Sampsons is exceedingly high, being higher than that of the poorest and most densely populated part of Liverpool.......'*

He was in no doubt as to the cause of this, suggesting *'The great cause for this mortality is undoubtedly improper feeding, and only those familiar with the ways of the poorer classes can realise how deeply rooted are their prejudices in this matter. The mistress of the situation is the elderly female friend or relation, and the more garrulous she is, and the greater number of children she has buried, the greater the authority she is reckoned to be in the bringing up of children.'*

He therefore recommended that *'Attempts are made to lower this mortality by the introduction of sterilised milk depots and early notification of the births, coupled with a visiting staff of ladies especially instructed in the preservation of the health of children.'*

In particular, he was a great enthusiast for the promotion of breastfeeding noting *'A healthy mother with breastmilk is free from noxious organisms, and a child will thrive on it better than any artificial food, and escape many serious and fatal infantile ailments, and thus grow up with a good foundation for the enjoyment of vigorous health throughout life'*. [MoH Report 1909]

He continued the theme some three years later *'Apart from other considerations, it is far cheaper for the mother to nurse the child if she is able, even if a quantity of excellent nourishment has to be given her. Breastmilk only is the natural food for babies during the first few months of life......'* [MoH Report 1912]

He later commented *'Upon doctors and nurses rests the responsibility of urging mothers to accept these duties. Perhaps both fail in some measure, but I am sorry to say that the advice of the doctor is often unheeded, because so many nurses are strongly unaccountably biased in favour of artificial feeding of infants. I believe the time will come when nurses who are licensed under the 'Midwives Act' and give such advice indiscriminately will be considered unfit persons to practice their calling, and will be treated as such.'* [MoH Report 1915]

An effort was made to start a 'Mothers Clinic' and Henry Draper Bishop reported *'An afternoon a week to be set aside for this purpose by the Medical Officer of Health. In spite of this being advertised, no one attended. This was a disappointing result.'* [MoH Report 1916]

He therefore called for the appointment of Health Visitors to address the continuing high infant mortality rate, but despite the *'invaluable work of the Infant and Nursing Associations in the Parishes, progress was slow.'* It was not until 1948 that two full-time paid Health Visitors were appointed.

High Maternal Deaths

Of as great concern as the high infant mortality was the unacceptable number of mothers dying in childbirth. Dr Henry Draper Bishop had noted in 1913 *'The statement that no arrangements are made here by the Parishes for the medical attention of poor women in labour will come as a shock to the public, as indeed it should. Of course it would be said that the health of the expectant mother should be looked after during her pregnancy, but how can this be achieved by ten separate parish authorities? The whole system of medical attendances for the poorer classes requires to be revised in a drastic fashion, and poor women in difficult labour ought to be able to secure immediate medical assistance in such a grave emergency'*. [MoH Report 1913]

The situation however continued to deteriorate. During the period 1908-1912, there had been ten maternal deaths, a rate of 1:493 births.

During the five years 1917-1921, there were to be twenty one maternal deaths, an increase to 1:175 births. Dr Henry Draper Bishop wrote.

'These are deeply disquieting statistics and the rapid increase in the number of these is so distressing, since in many instances these are preventable deaths...... it is therefore to me a matter of great regret that my suggestions for the registration, training and control of Midwives was not taken up by the Board of Health, the Board being of the opinion that if legislation was really necessary, the question should be submitted to the States by the Parochial Authorities or other bodies interested in infant welfare.'

Action was eventually forced by the outcry of 1933 when nine maternal deaths were recorded in a single year - a rate of 1:79 births. Dr Henry Draper Bishop was moved to comment *'This is the most distressing figure that I ever had to give in my 33 years experience here ...... there is no obligation on the part of the doctor of midwife in attendance to report such deaths to the Medical Officer of Health, and in most instances I had no knowledge of them until some time had elapsed.'*

Whilst conducting the inquest into the cause of death of one unfortunate young married woman during childbirth, the magistrate *'had expressed great surprise that although physicians and surgeons no matter how well qualified are not permitted to practice in the island without first obtaining permission from the Royal Court, anyone qualified or not can practice as a Midwife'.*

H M Comptroller duly wrote to the Board of Health *'asking them to consider what steps should be taken to ensure that in future the lives of mothers on the island may not be endangered as a result of erroneous treatment by unqualified midwives'.*

Under such pressure, the States reacted quickly and a *'Midwives Act'* was proposed in 1934 and came into effect on 1st October 1936. Dr Henry Draper Bishop was able to comment *'This should have a considerable effect in raising the level of midwifery amongst the poorer mothers on the island, as it enables Midwives to call on medical assistance when available, even though the mother is unable to pay the fees.'*

Regular returns of emergency medical attention required during labour became a standard inclusion in the Annual MoH Reports for many years afterwards, and over twenty years later it was still being reported that medical aid was given free of charge to 117 *'necessitous mothers'* in 1958, and to a further 146 similar cases in 1959.

Influenza epidemic 1918-1919

In the first decades if this century, infectious diseases were a common cause of death, being responsible for around one hundred and eighty deaths annually, or around one quarter of all deaths recorded. In addition, there were periodic epidemics, such as the pandemic of 'Spanish Influenza' which swept across Europe in the aftermath of the First World War.

There had only been eight deaths recorded as being due to influenza in the period 1906-1916. In 1917 there were nine such deaths, and in 1918 one hundred and fifteen deaths felt to be due to influenza and its complications.

In October a special meeting of the Board of Health was called to consider the situation, and in view of the urgency of the matter, it was decided to refer it to the Royal Court.

The Royal Court met especially on 26th October 1918, and upon the advice of the Board of Health agreed to immediately close all schools, places of public entertainment and to prohibit all unofficial gatherings of people.

The Board published warning notices in the newspapers and posters in both French and English, which were exhibited throughout the island suggesting the precautions against infection which should be taken. The use of 'Thalasol' (a strong disinfectant manufactured from seawater by a special plant located on the Careening Hard in St Peter Port) was advocated as a gargle and nasal douche, and supplies of it were distributed freely throughout the island.

The Sanatorium was also made available for severe cases which could not be nursed at home. Despite these measures, there was a re-occurrence of influenza in the early months of 1919, which caused a further forty deaths, twenty six of which were in people aged between 25 and 65.

Dr Henry Draper Bishop had his own views regarding the spread of infection;

'The visiting of sick people is a constant feature of our community where close relations are so common .... many people unfortunately lost their lives as a result of such visiting. A proportion of the deaths were those of young adults and people in the prime of life'.

The 1918-1919 influenza pandemic is said to have been responsible for twenty million deaths world wide - more fatalities than suffered by all combatants during World War One. The 115 influenza related civilian deaths in just two winters in Guernsey compares with the 327 officers and men of the Royal Guernsey Light Infantry who lost their lives in France during the Great War.

Tackling other infectious diseases

The appointment of a Medical Officer of Health in Guernsey and the establishment of the Board of Health are linked to the outbreak of diphtheria at the turn of the century. But although the original outbreak was quickly brought under control, further epidemics continued to occur in the following decades. There was a particularly bad outbreak in 1938, with 489 cases of infection and 14 deaths, mainly in children and young adults.

A more effective response than the traditional measures of isolating cases and disinfecting premises was obviously required, and voluntary immunisation against diphtheria was therefore proposed. However, uptake of immunisation on a voluntary basis was insufficient, and a Projet de Loi entitled *'L'inoculation des enfants contra la diphtherie'* was considered and passed by the States on 24th June 1938.

All children between the ages of 2 and 10 years were required to attend for free immunisation, and attempts were made by means of notices in newspapers and distribution of pamphlets through schools to persuade as many parents as possible to have their children inoculated. This quickly proved effective, and the then Medical Officer of Health Dr Rowan Revell wrote *'Without inoculation, no such marked fall would have been expected before the end of March or in April.'*

In 1939 there was a resurgence of diphtheria, but with fewer than two hundred cases and four deaths. Dr Rowan Revell commented *'When diphtheria is not prevalent, it is very difficult to persuade parents to have their children inoculated, but to prevent future epidemics of this disease, it is essential to maintain a high percentage of inoculated children and in my opinion, this can only be effected by some sort of compulsion, such as is now in force in the island.'*

Although cases continued to occur until the early 1950's there was never again to be a major epidemic of diphtheria. For those generations of Guernsey children born since this time, diphtheria must now seem as unlikely a cause of disease or death as the 'black death' or 'great plague'.

The control of tuberculosis

In parallel with the control of diphtheria comes the fall in other infectious diseases. By far the most feared of these was tuberculosis, sometimes described in earlier medical textbooks as the *'great white plague'*.

In 1903, the then MoH Dr Henry Draper-Bishop wrote *'One out of every six deaths must be attributed to tuberculosis, a disease, which under ideal conditions, is preventable ...... amongst the predisposing causes of the disease are overcrowding, intemperance, deficiency of food, dampness of houses and soil, insufficient and impure air, exposure to rapid alterations of temperature, sedentary occupations, especially those requiring cramped positions and as a sequel to other illnesses .... the filthy habit of indiscriminate spitting should be prohibited by law as is now done in other places'.*

Tuberculosis remained a significant cause of death until after World War Two, but declined dramatically following this. Improvements in housing, nutrition and general social conditions undoubtedly contributed towards this, as did health measures such as the opening of the States Sanatorium, advances in anti-tuberculosis therapy and the surgical treatment of cavitational lesions, combined with public health responses which included mass radiography and the scrupulous 'contact tracing' of family and social contacts of new 'index' cases.

When he retired in 1983, Guernsey's seventh MoH Dr Geoffrey White was able to write *'The greatest single change in the past twenty years has been the reduction in the incidence of tuberculosis'*.

'..........One of my first tasks in 1962 was to accept responsibility for the two wards of cases of pulmonary tuberculosis at the King Edward Sanatorium: between 15 and 20 cases in each ward, where men and women languished for months rather than weeks whilst their lungs healed sufficiently that they were no longer an infectious risk and so could circulate in the community once more .... nowadays the Sanatorium has ceased to function as an infectious diseases hospital, and nowhere else is a single bed allocated specifically for the treatment of TB'.

The smoking epidemic

Public health legislation has slowly brought environmental hazards to health under control, whilst immunisation and therapeutic advances have largely banished previous patterns of disease and death from infectious disease. Improved obstetric care, the appointment of Health Visitors and the promotion of breastfeeding, together with a general rise in standards of living have reduced infant mortality to a fraction of what it was at the turn of the century.

However, whilst many causes of death have declined, some newer epidemics still await to be effectively tackled, high amongst which is the current epidemic of smoking related disease.

As long ago as 1909 Dr Henry Draper Bishop had commented *'The rate of damage to young people by the abuse of cigarettes is clearly shown by the Army Medical Department. ... who found that no less than 30% of the recruits examined for the Army between 1906 and 1907 were rejected on account of diseases of the heart ...... it is considered by many that the cigarette habit of recent years has played an important part in causing this most frequent occurrence of functional disease of the heart. Average British recruits are on enlistment in the poorest physical condition of those in any civilised army. Moreover they are nearly all confirmed cigarette smokers.'*

A 1913 Ordinance prohibiting the gift or sale of tobacco and cigarettes to persons under the age of 16 was described as *'a most useful one'*, and it was later remarked *'In the opinion of those best qualified to judge, it appears to have worked extremely well, which is more than perhaps than was generally expected when it was first passed.'*

However, smoking levels continued to rise amongst the adult population, and with it the burden of lung cancer and other smoking related diseases. In 1960, the then MoH Dr A Thomas pointed out that the lung cancer rate had risen from 8 per year in 1951 to 25 per year in 1958. *'It has been generally agreed that a special effort should be directed at encouraging young people not to start smoking, but this is a great deal easier said than done'* he wrote.

A joint Committee was established between Guernsey, Jersey and Alderney in 1977 *'for the declared aim of reducing cigarette consumption throughout the Channel Islands - in response to the high mortality from cigarette related disease which is the experience of the Island population.'* Warnings on cigarette packages were introduced as a result.

By the early 1990's is was calculated that between 100 and 130 Guernsey residents died each year from smoking related disease, about half of them prematurely. Using such compelling evidence, in 1996 the Board of Health was finally able to persuade the States to bring in a comprehensive range of measures designed to make smoking less attractive, less accessible and less affordable to young people, and to offer practical help to addicted adult smokers who wished to quit.

This package of measures included local bans on tobacco advertising, raising tobacco prices steadily over a six year period, raising the legal age of purchase from 16 to 18 years, providing special school and community based programmes warning of the dangers of smoking, and offering additional assistance to addicted smokers who wished to stop. At the time, the British Medical Journal reported this as *'the most important precedent in tobacco control in the western world in recent years'*.

Building on the public health successes of the past century, the future role of the Medical Officer of Health must be to continue gather robust information on those changing factors which may adversely affect the health of the population, and to devise and implement effective strategies to tackle and control these.

Although the focus may change, providing the underlying principles of public health are maintained, there is no reason why present trends towards increased longevity and better health well into old age in both Guernsey and Alderney should not continue well into the next Millennium.

Main Sources;

- Annual Reports of the Medical Officer of Health for Guernsey: 1899-1998
- Minutes of the Board of Health: 1900-1903; 1932-1938
- Guernsey Star: 1899
- Guernsey Evening Press - various dates

Note

This chapter is based in part on an address given to La Société Guernesiaise on 26th March 1996, a summary of which appeared in the *'La Société Guernesiaise - Report and Transactions 1995'* Volume XXIII. V; 964-72.

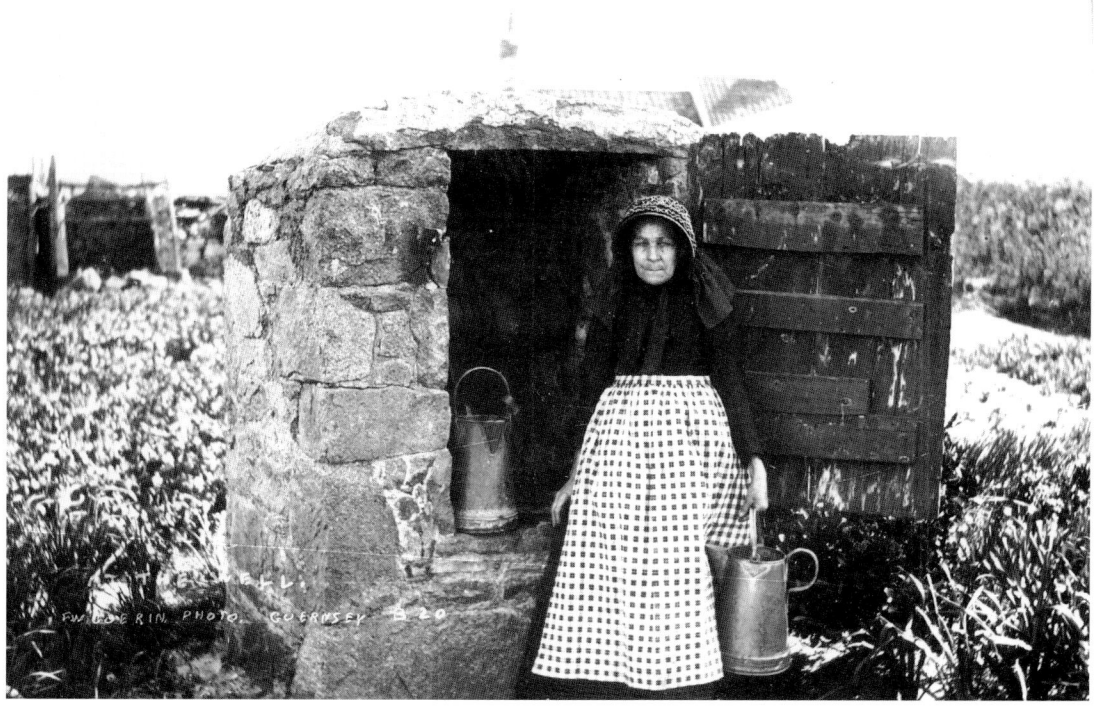

Collecting Water - around 1900   G0380

'The chief source of danger to public health in Guernsey consists of the unsatisfactory construction of the closets, pig sties, etc and the close proximity of wells to such sources of pollution .... Dirty water when used to cleanse milk utensils cannot leave them in a clean state ...... that milk is one of the chief means of spring diarrhoea is evidenced by the fact that infants under a year form the chief victims of the attack.

There is a great necessity that some ordinances should be passed regulating their construction ...... until such legal matters are taken, it would be almost impossible to effect improvement in the sanitation of Guernsey'.

Annual Report of the Medical Office of Health 1899

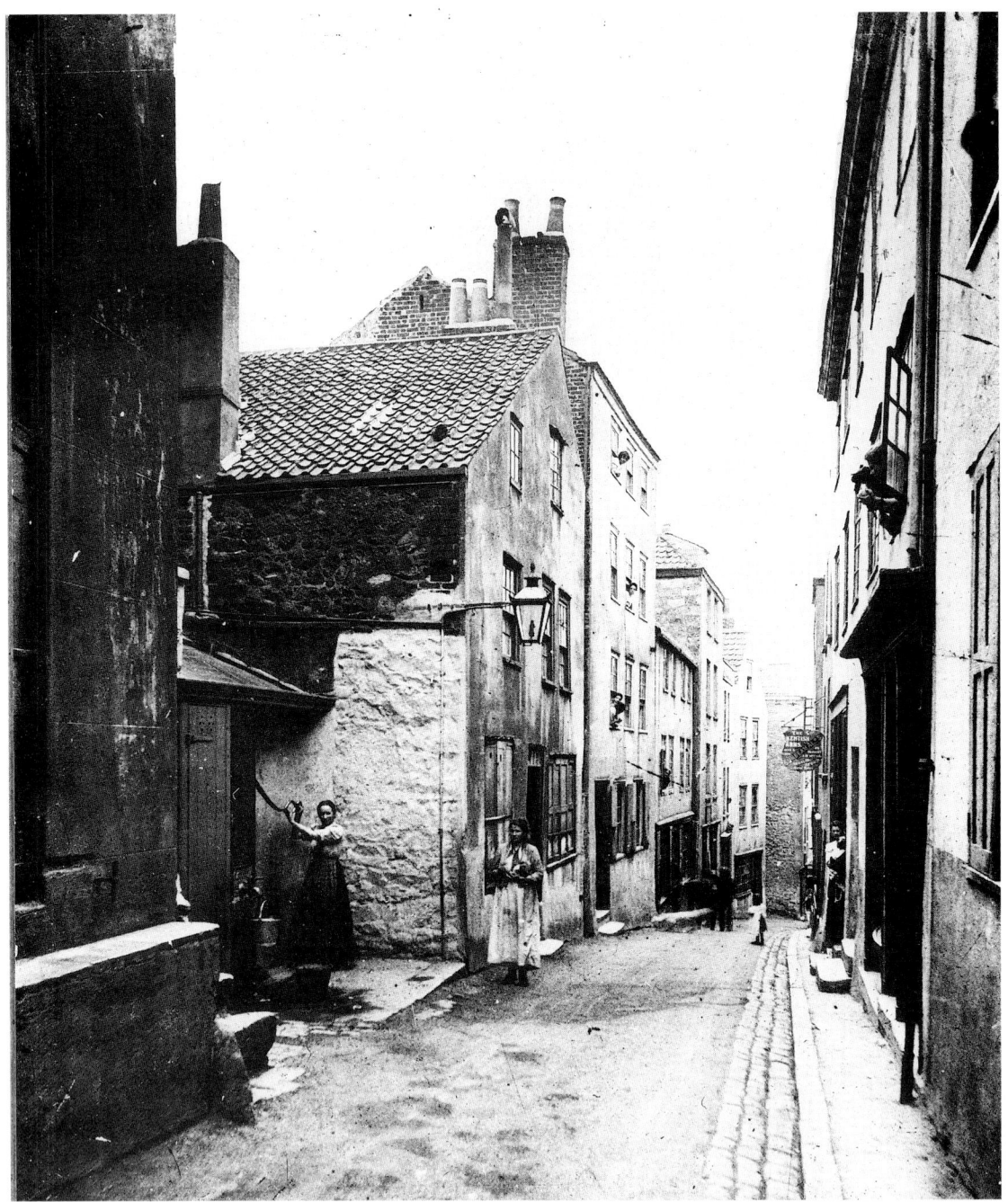

Public pump in Cornet Street around 1900   G0094

'A large number of houses in the town rely upon the public pumps for all purposes. As the wells are fairly deep the pumps are hard to work and women and children in addition to pumping water have to carry it long distances, often up flights of stairs to the houses and tenements. It is no wonder then that dirty houses and badly flushed drains cause disease amongst the population so scantily supplied with one of the necessities of life. To add to the difficulties of these unfortunate people, some of these pumps have in the summer run dry'.

Annual Report of the Medical Office of Health 1911

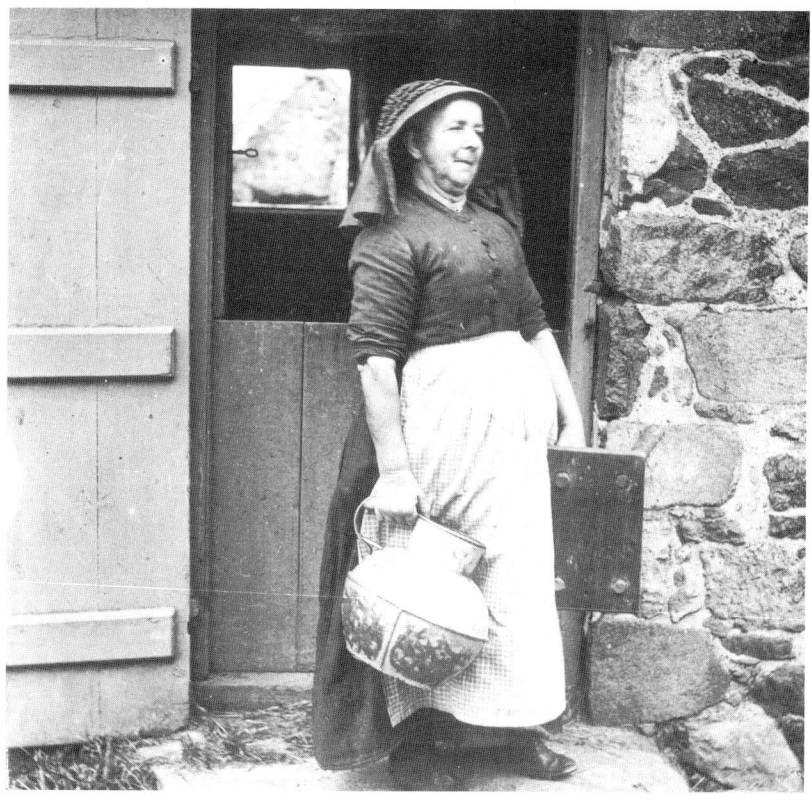

Collecting milk in a Guernsey can G0381

'For the past twenty five years I have been endeavouring to get a standard fixed for Guernsey milk, and not having been successful have used the English standard for purpose of analysis, although for our milk it is much too low.

This procedure has not been challenged until this year, when a farmer was produced before the Police Court for selling milk adulterated with water. The case was dismissed by the magistrate, who stated as there was no recognised standard for Guernsey milk, there could be no conviction. The public therefore have no protection against the dishonest milk vendor'.

Annual Report of the Medical Officer of Health 1933

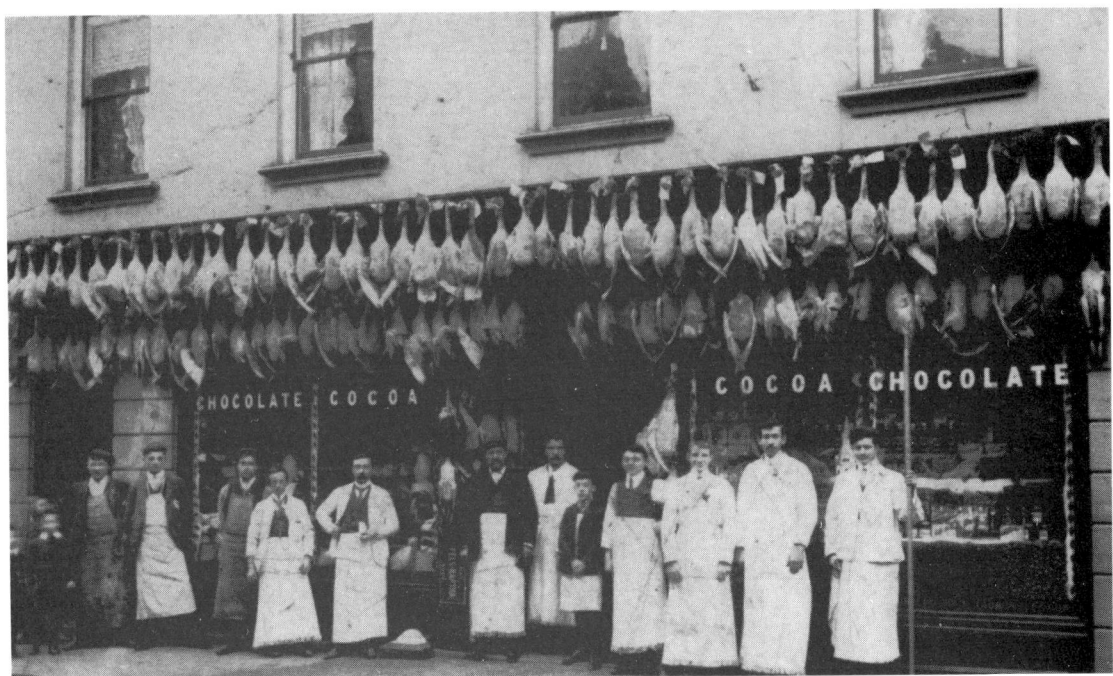

Guernsey Grocery shop around 1910

'Public concerns regarding the safety of food have increased despite local food hygiene standards being raised. The sensationalisation of food issues at various times by the media has led to waves of frequently unfounded anxieties amongst the public'. (Chapter Two)

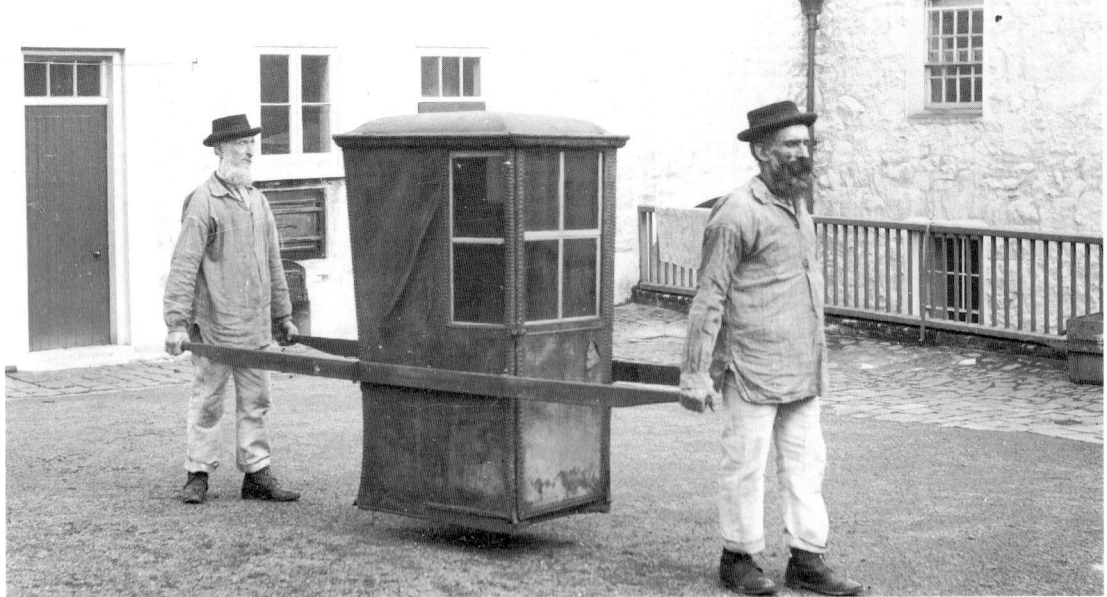

Sedan Chair   G0387

'For many years the Town Hospital hired out a sedan chair for people who wished to travel short distances around the town, and the inmates carried this'. (Chapter Three)

Chapter Two

From sanitary reform to planetary protection

John Cook

At the turn of the century, responsibility for sanitation and refuse disposal was firmly vested in the Douzaines and their Parish Constables - powers they were reluctant to surrender. It took 36 years to achieve a uniform approach to environmental health throughout the island, and a further 30 years before the legal armamentarium *necessary to ensure environmental safety was reasonably complete. In the final one third of the century, environmental concerns have of necessity become far more global.*

Sanitary reform

The background to the development of Public Health in Guernsey at the end of the nineteenth century can be found in events which occurred in Britain almost a century beforehand - particularly the conditions which were allowed to develop as a result of the Industrial Revolution.

Manufacturing centres had became established and as a consequence large industrial towns had grown up. These towns lacked the amenities and infrastructure to adequately support the large numbers of workers and their families who migrated there, attracted by such advertisements as: "*To families desirous of settling in Macclesfield: Wanted four to five thousand people between the age of 7 and 21.*" (Cheshire Newspaper Early 19th Century)

Industrial pollution, poor housing, overcrowding, inadequate sanitation and contaminated water supplies were all common. Disease and early death amongst the working classes became a public concern. This concern heightened when it became clear that disease, whilst most prevalent amongst the poor, recognised no social barriers and epidemics could affect all sectors of society.

A series of Royal Commissions were established which reported to Parliament on the dire sanitary conditions of the "labouring population of Great Britain".

The resulting Public Health Bill became, after much debate and delay, particularly at the committee stage, Britain's first *Public Health Act* in 1848.

This Act established a General Board of Health and allowed for the introduction of Local Boards.

The genesis of sanitary reform was thus established. Local Boards of Health were to appoint a qualified medical practitioner as Medical Officer of Health and *'fit and proper persons'* to be Inspectors of Nuisances. The recognised environmental hazards of pollution, offensive trades, housing and insanitary conditions were able to be systematically addressed for the first time.

At this stage, however, only 183 local Boards of Health were established covering 3 million people out of a total population in Britain of 27 million. London and all of Scotland were excluded from the provisions of the Act.

For the next quarter of a century legislation supporting the sanitary ideal continued to occupy the attention of Parliament. The *Nuisances Removal and Disease Prevention Act* was passed in 1855, and the *Sanitary Act* in 1866. Inspectors of Nuisances were obligatory appointments and were referred to as Sanitary Inspectors for the first time.

The *Public Health Act* of 1875 consolidated the whole of the patchwork of the Public Health Law in Great Britain and justly earned the sobriquet the *'Great Charter of Public Health'*.

Environmental hazards in Guernsey

Guernsey was largely unaffected by the Industrial Revolution. In the second half of the nineteenth century horticulture, agriculture and the quarrying of granite were the mainstays of the Island's economy, with summer visitors becoming increasingly common.

Whilst avoiding the trend to concentrate populations of workers, there were, nevertheless, concerns over sanitary standards. Ordinances were introduced in the 1850s and 60s which dealt with the condition of drains, latrines and cesspits in St Peter Port. In an Ordinance of 1853, whose preamble referred to the spread of cholera and the rules in force in England at the time, the first reference was made to statutory public health nuisances.

The nuisances referred to specifically included ditches, latrines, cesspits, piles of rubbish and animals kept in such a manner as to be a nuisance or prejudicial to public health, and even any house which was a nuisance or prejudicial to public health by reason of its dirty or unhealthy condition. This provision was repeated in subsequent Ordinances. The controls were available to the St Peter Port Parochial Authorities only but gradually extended to those of other parishes with the powers firmly residing with Douzaines and Parish Constables. In 1866 a fairly clumsy procedure to deal with overcrowding was proposed whilst detailed provisions dealing specifically with infectious diseases were enacted in subsequent years together with a piecemeal strengthening of other aspects of the Ordinances.

How an outbreak and continuance of diphtheria in Guernsey at the end of the last century ultimately led to the appointment of the first Medical Officer of Health and the establishment of the Board of Health have already been described in Chapter One.

Whilst primarily concerned with the measures necessary to control this outbreak of diphtheria, Guernsey's first Medical Officer of Health Dr John Brownlea was quick to comment on other issues such as public health nuisance and environmental pollution.

In his first Annual Report (1899) he noted *"There is a knackery however on the Banques which I was requested by the Constable of St Sampson's Parish to visit and report upon. The methods pursued at this knackery are such as are calculated to produce the maximum of nuisance."* He called for regulation of all such offensive trades.

"I think that the matter is of sufficient importance to demand a special report with the view to the regulation of such trades as soap boiling, manure manufacturing, &c., by Ordinance of the Royal Court.'

He also, perhaps more significantly, made reference to the link between unsatisfactory closets, pigsties etc, polluted water, the cross contamination of milk and the high incidence of diarrhoea in the Island. He evoked that *"Until some legal measures are taken, it will be almost impossible to effect improvement in the sanitation of Guernsey, for it must be perfectly evident, that with the legal disabilities at present in force, that a prosecution is so difficult a matter as to preclude any recourse to it, except in some glaring instance of infraction of the law.'*

Although originally appointed only for a period *"up to three years"* Dr Brownlea decided to leave Guernsey after little more than one year, to take up the post of Physician Superintendent at the Glasgow Fever Hospital. Dr E Stanley Hoare was appointed in his place, and in the second annual report of the Medical Officer of Health, (1900) he called for the appointment of an official 'Sanitary Inspector'.

This call must have been answered, since Guernsey's third Medical Officer of Health Dr Henry Draper Bishop, writing in the Annual Report for 1903 lists the work completed by Mr Le Brun as Sanitary Inspector. His works would appear to have consisted of the disinfection of various articles, bed linen, rooms and schools associated with outbreaks of infectious disease. As Draper Bishop was later to remark (1913) *'At present the position of Sanitary Inspector is not recognised by law, and but few duties can be assigned to him'*.

Dr Draper Bishop had in an earlier Report (1909), commented on the disadvantages of having each Douzaine acting as an independent Sanitary Authority *"Many of the public health laws in force in Guernsey were passed before the formation of the board of Health, therefore sanitary administration continues in great measure to be still carried out by the Douzaines. I think the time has now arrived when the Board of Health should be invested with more powers and responsibilities"*.

From this point until 1934 the Medical Officer of Health's reports contained repeated calls for improvements to the Laws protecting Public Health and for increased powers for the Medical Officer of Health and Sanitary Inspector.

Public health protection

Basic sanitary problems persisted. Housing, sewerage and refuse collection and disposal issues all featured; as did the contamination of drinking water and milk, and the adulteration of food.

Other issues appear to have had more significance at that time than currently. In his 1924 annual report Dr Draper Bishop strongly advocated the prohibition of night baking but, as history would suggest, to little avail. *"The making of bread during the night is now prohibited in many countries. I know of no reason why it should be permitted in England and Guernsey, and I trust it will not be for much longer. Not only is bread likely to be made under unsatisfactory and uncleanly conditions at night by artificial light, but it is inhumane and uneconomic to make men continually work by night instead of by day as Nature intended, unless such work be absolutely* necessary."

In response to Dr Draper Bishop's years of prompting, the States finally agreed to the *Loi Relative de la Sante Publique* in 1934, the year of Dr Draper Bishop's retirement at the age of 70 years, after over 33 years as Guernsey's Medical Officer of Health.

This new Law, which was firmly rooted in the 'Great' Public Health Act of 1875, empowered the Medical Officer of Health and Sanitary Inspector to gain entry to premises Island-wide and to require the abatement of specific conditions deemed to be injurious to health or a nuisance.

Housing conditions, water pollution, the accumulation of refuse, the condition of workplaces and the noise, vibration and smoke arising from workplaces were also addressed.

The introduction of the *Ordinance Provisional a la Sante Publique* in 1936 gave added powers and penalties in relation to Public Health nuisances and included provisions relating to the notification of disease, the prevention of spread of infection, the inspection of farms and dairies and emergency powers.

Guernsey, at last, had produced its own "Charter of Public Health" and issues of direct public health concern could thus be more effectively tackled. Public Health protection became the aim rather than the limited sanitary view of merely preventing the spread of disease.

The effects of the Occupation

The advent of the Second World War, the partial evacuation of Guernsey and the Occupation of the Island by German troops and migrant workers led to a severe regression in public health standards.

Guernsey's fourth Medical Officer of Health Dr. Rowan Revell, together with his long serving Senior States Sanitary Inspector Mr George Austin and Sanitary Assistants struggled to maintain standards of public health despite increasing shortages of materials and labour, and the deterioration of sanitary facilities.

Properties occupied by migrant workers and troops were reported as overcrowded, filthy and verminous with inadequate sanitary arrangements - almost an echo of the worst conditions of the Industrial Revolution half a century before in England. It is a bitter irony that having only relatively recently introduced legislation based upon 1875 United Kingdom standards, Guernsey should be faced with conditions reminiscent of this earlier era.

The health of Guernsey during the Occupation is further considered in Chapter Nine. The cessation of the War led to a period of rebuilding and consolidation rather than a continuation of pre-war developments in public health.

The abatement of statutory nuisances that affected the health and well-being of individuals or groups was at the core of the Public Health Services in Guernsey. However, overcrowding and poor housing conditions proved difficult to alleviate at a time of material shortages.

Progress in food legislation

Good standards of food hygiene were difficult to enforce and the Chief Sanitary Inspector and the Medical Officer of Health made repeated requests between 1950 and 1970 for legislation to be introduced to control the production and sale of food.

Dr A Thomas, Guernsey fourth Medical Officer of Health, reported in his 1963 Annual Report *'During 1963 some progress was made towards legal rearmament of the Public Health Department, but it is a slow business. It seems most desirable, if not ultimately inevitable, that the main provisions of the Food and Drugs Act of 1955 should be adopted in the Island, and indeed, this matter is far advanced in Jersey.'*

It took until 1970, however, for the *Food and Drugs (Guernsey)* Law to be introduced.

In the meanwhile in 1964, Mr George Austin the long serving Chief Sanitary Inspector retired and was replaced by Mr John Ball, as Chief Public Health Inspector. Mr Ball was a UK qualified Public Health Inspector and the change of title and the move to UK trained personnel is, perhaps, a significant indication of a strategic move from sanitary reforms to broader public health protection, a move which was aimed at correcting those conditions that have a direct deleterious effect on the physical health of the public.

The *Food and Drugs (Guernsey) Law,* 1970 and subsequent *Food and Drugs (Food Hygiene) Order* 1976 were eventually introduced, mirroring UK legislation of 1955 and 1970.

For a while it was felt that the Public Health Department had adequate legislative powers to protect the physical health of the local public from adverse local circumstances .

Although it was felt food safety could be controlled at a local level, patterns in food production and distribution continued to evolve and change. Large scale, centralised food production and manufacture, together with expanding international distribution meant that food safety problems experienced in one region or country might have effects world-wide.

Since Guernsey now imports a large majority of its food, it could not avoid being affected by food safety issues beyond its local control.

Public concerns regarding the safety of food have increased despite local food hygiene standards being raised. The sensationalisation of food issues at various times by the media has led to waves of frequently unfounded anxieties amongst the public.

Dubious historic doubts regarding night-time baking are being superseded by global food scares.

As the century ends, the spectre of a whole nations beef industry being destroyed by one pathogen (Bovine Spongiform Encephalopathy) and a huge section of another nations food output being recalled from around the world due to contamination (Dioxin) places the relevance of food protection at a local level in a wider perspective.

Environmental Concern

In 1979, John Ball retired as Chief Public Health Inspector and was replace by Mr Mike Bairds. In his first annual report Mr Bairds made reference to growing concerns of threats to the environment being a public health issue. *"As rapid advances in science and technology put ever increasing strain on the environment, the range and complexities of complaints and routine work naturally expands due to increasing public awareness and concern."*

His comment serves to illustrate the rapidly developing international awareness that long term damage was being inflicted upon the global environment. At this time there was also a steadily increasing understanding of the effect of environmental factors on health, and the individuals ability to sustain it.

A number of well reported international commissions and conferences have attempted to address this issue, most significant were the World Commission on Environment and Development (WCED) 1987, The International Panel on Climate Change (IPCC) 1990 and the United Nations Conference on the Environment and Development ('Earth Summit') Rio de Janeiro 1992.

It is now widely accepted that man's activities are having an increasingly adverse effect on the global environment, which in turn is posing increasing risks to sustainable human health around the world. Such risks to health cannot be resolved in isolation, but require co-ordinated international action.

Public health, therefore, is increasingly being linked to environmental conditions which, long-term, cannot be resolved by local, retrospective, legal action; the basis of Guernsey's public health controls.

The World Health Organisation (WHO) has defined environmental health as being *"the control of all those factors in man's physical environment which exercise, or may exercise, a deleterious effect on his physical development, health or survival'*. In this context, health is said to mean: *'a state of complete physical, mental and social well being'*.

Environmental health, therefore, is a broad concept but one which is, nevertheless, only one facet of public health. According to the 1992 Government White Paper *'The Health of the Nation' 'Public health is the science and art of preventing disease, prolonging life and promoting health through the organised efforts of society'*.

In 1983, in response to their widening environmental role, Guernsey's Public Health Inspectors were recognised as Environmental Health Officers.

The departments environmental protection involvement has expanded and old sanitary reform measures and nuisance abatement measures available have became increasingly inadequate. Long-term measures to prevent the activities of Guernsey's population from contributing to adverse global effects were recognised as being necessary. On Wednesday 26th February 1997 the States of Guernsey approved Board of Health proposals for a *'Control of Environmental Pollution Law'*. In the same Billet d'Etat the *'Loi Relative de la Sante Publique,'* 1934 and Ordinance of 1936 were amended.

The *'Control of Environmental Pollution'* Law includes provision to prevent environmental pollution by controlling waste disposal, discharges to sea, discharges to air and the generation of noise. The Billet reflected a philosophy of 'prevention rather than cure' as follows:

"Whilst the proposals outlined in the above paragraph of this report will enable the Board to act effectively against public health nuisances, the Board is of the opinion that new legislative provisions are needed which, rather than rectifying existing nuisances, enable control measures to be placed on those activities which present a risk of pollution.

In order to protect the environment and those resources which are an essential prerequisite to good health, a proactive integrated approach, which protects the environment from harm, is essential.

The general thrust of the proposed new Law is, therefore, proactive rather than reactive and this general policy of prevention rather than cure is reflected in proposals that require prior consent and/or licences to he obtained before potentially polluting activities are undertaken. The proposals recognise that, as far as is practicable, an integrated approach is required to control environmental pollution, with systems that are designed to prevent pollution rather than to deal with pollution once it has occurred. This is not only beneficial for the environment but has the added advantage of being a much more efficient and effective use of the expertise available within the Environmental Health Department, whose officers would administer the legislation on behalf of the Board.

Although this law has not been finally enacted as we reach the Board of Health's first centenary, the direction is clear and Environmental Health Officers in Guernsey will begin the second century with a broad remit and advancing technological capacity to protect people, their health, their well-being and their quality of existence. There is now an intent to maintain established international environmental standards and share in global responsibility.

Bad housing, infectious disease, insanitary conditions and unsound food will continue to be an immediate threat that cannot be ignored, but now of equal importance is the need to ensure that our global environment is maintained so as also to give future generations equal opportunity for good health and continuing well-being.

As appreciation of man's role in the global environment expands, and understanding of our mutual responsibility to preserve the ecosystem we inhabit increases, so Environmental Health criteria and priorities will continue to evolve.

The *'fit and proper persons'* employed as Inspectors of Nuisances and Sanitary Inspectors in Guernsey during the past century are now being replaced by M.Sc. Graduates, who are also members of the Chartered Institute of Environmental Health.

In 100 years, the environmental health perspective has swung from disinfecting after infection to prevent spread, through the improvement of physical conditions intended to prevent future outbreak, to the urgent need to help preserve a viable environment to sustain generations yet to come.

It is a challenge still to be met.

Chapter Three

The story of the Town Hospital 1900-1987

Gillian Lenfestey

When the Board of Health first met in 1900, the Town Hospital had already existed for over 150 years. Although it was to remain independent of the Board until 1970, it never quite lived down the stigma of its origins, having once been a poorhouse. Its few remaining patients were finally transferred to other accommodation in October 1986.

'House of Charity'

When the Board of Health was officially constituted in December 1899 the Town Hospital had already been in existence for over one hundred and fifty years. Built in 1742, originally as a House of Charity for the poor of the town and parish of St Peter Port it was soon also used as an orphanage, a maternity and medical hospital and a night-stay unit for drunks.

It was administered initially by a committee comprising a Treasurer and Directors elected by the Parish, with the Constables, Procureur of the Poor, Rector and Churchwardens as ex officio members. By the end of the 19th century it came under the control of the Poor Law Board with a Hospital Board or House Committee which dealt with the day to day running of the establishment. The employees consisted of a Matron and Master (who were often husband and wife), a second Matron and Master, cook, labour master, and various tradesmen, for example a plumber and a shoemaker.

Facilities also existed at the Town Hospital for parishioners who did not live at the Hospital to receive medical treatment. A public Dispensary had been opened in 1853 and the parish had retained a doctor to treat the 'outdoor' poor since the 1750s. The doctor could be requested by one of the Overseers of the Poor to visit the sick in their own homes, or the patient could be asked to visit the doctor at his surgery at the Town Hospital. This was a single storey building in the south-east corner of the Hospital yard, consisting of a waiting room and two small surgeries. If the patient was given a prescription they could have it made up at the Dispensary, which was in a room diagonally across the yard underneath the archway which linked the two main buildings.

The turn of the century

By 1900 the workhouse occupied the ground floor of the Old Building, the basements, and buildings in the back yard. The medical side of the establishment (usually called the Infirmary) used the first and second floors in the Old Building, and the first floor in the New Building. It was run by a qualified nursing sister and two qualified nurses, with unqualified assistants. However the Master of the Town Hospital was in overall charge.

The care of the poor was traditionally a parish responsibility using funds levied on the parishioners. Each parish had its own Poor Law Board which administered the Poor Law through the Procureurs of the Poor who were elected by the parish. The Town Hospital, and later the Lunatic Asylum, were built specifically for the use of those domiciled in the town and parish of St Peter Port. If anyone else used the facilities their parish was invoiced accordingly. However the day to day running of the Town Hospital had always been overseen by a Hospital Committee which reported to the parochial Poor Law Board.

In 1902 the House Committee consisted of the vice-president of the Poor Law Board, one of the Constables of St Peter Port, the Procureur of the Poor, three Overseers and a former member of the Board. Their remit included not only the Workhouse, but also the Infirmary, the Lunatic Asylum and the Children's Home which did not yet have buildings of its own. They were responsible for the employment of staff, capital expenditure of any kind, alterations and improvements of any kind, the application of new Laws, and so forth. However all their decisions had to be ratified by the Poor Law Board.

This situation changed after the First World War. In 1925 a new Poor Law was passed which transferred the cost of Poor Law Administration from the parishes to the States. A Central Board was set up which was assisted by Boards in each of the parishes, and one for the Country Hospital. The St Peter Port Board also administered the Town Hospital. Then in 1937 the functions of all these Boards were transferred to the States Public Assistance Authority and a Hospital Board was formed which was responsible for all the hospitals. Poor Relief, or Public Assistance as it is now called, is still administered under the 1937 Law, as amended.

Other people also became involved in the care of the poor and one of the better known of these was Mrs Margaret Neve. On her death in 1903 the Poor Law Board expressed their condolences to her nephew, Col. Harvey, who was Vice-President at the time, saying that she had always given ready help to cases of distress, and how much they had appreciated her inviting the Hospital children to picnics at her house during haymaking time.

In 1905 it was suggested that the Town Hospital be sold to the States. The Poor Law Board referred the matter to the ratepayers of St Peter Port, to whom the place belonged, and following a meeting of the States Committee on Poor Law Administration various proposals were made. A Lunatic Asylum was to be provided for the whole island, under a separate administration; a central committee was to be appointed to administer the Infirmary and the Workhouse; that these should be separate from each other, and only one of each should exist on the island; the children should be kept separate from either of the above. The funds for carrying out these schemes should be provided partly by the States and partly by ratepayers.

The States pointed out that if the ratepayers refused to sell and the States found the properties unsuitable they could decide to put up other buildings for the carrying out of the scheme, and the ratepayers would be saddled with useless buildings, and would also have to contribute to the cost of the new buildings.

In view of this, on 22 December 1905 the ratepayers resolved to sell to the States the buildings and land of the Hospital, and the buildings and land of the Lunatic Asylum. The price would be fixed by expert estimate, and the contents of the buildings would be included in the price. The significance of this was that the financial responsibility for the maintenance and upkeep of the establishment passed from the parish of St Peter Port to the States.

People were admitted to the Town Hospital for all sorts of reasons. Sometimes, like the Widow M, they were destitute. Sometimes, like Mrs A they were going blind and could no longer cope, and their children were also admitted. Mr P was brought in suffering from fits, and Sophie R. had whooping cough.

Apart from the regular maintenance of the building, for example 12 invalid beds with mattresses bought for £2.10s. each, the china at the Lunatic Asylum replaced with enamel ware, Leale's tender for £51.15s.6d for supplying and fixing a boiler and apparatus accepted, the item which stands out in the years before the First World War is the considerable turnover of staff at the Infirmary and Asylum.

The nurses and assistants come and go with almost alarming regularity. Also actions which would merely attract a reprimand nowadays were considered grounds for dismissal 90 years ago.

World War One

During the War arrangements were made to receive sick and wounded men of the Guernsey Militia should the occasion arise, and V.A.D's were allowed to work at the Hospital in order to gain practical experience.

In 1915 the House Committee considered offering a more valuable form of qualifying certificate to the assistant nurses, after a suitable examination. It was agreed that the doctors would give lectures in certain subjects and Sister would demonstrate the practical side of nursing. All the assistant nurses had to attend all the lectures and sit examinations at the end of each term. At the end of 3 years a certificate was given to those who had passed.

It was also decided at this time that the fully certificated superintendent nurse, who was now called Sister, should have full control of the nursing arrangements. The Master, Matron and 2nd Matron should be responsible for the able bodied inmates, and Sister should be responsible for the sick and infirm.

What life was like between the Wars

A note on salaries at the end of the First World War shows that the Master received £150 per year, and Matron £56. Sister received £77.10, and the qualified nurse £25. The Hospital tailor received £1.16.0d per week, the shoemaker £1.15.0d, and the laundress £1.

Various inmates received from 5/- to 1/6d per month. However the tailor's pay differed from week to week, and may have depended on how much clothing he made, or how many hours he worked.

In March 1920 as a result of various allegations having been made, there was an inquiry into unrest amongst the nursing staff. It would appear that the Master and Sister did not agree, and Dr Bisson recommended that the administration of the Infirmary and Workhouse be separated, with Sister reporting to the chairman of the House Committee rather than the Master.

In December 1920, in a letter to Mr de la Haye at the Jersey General Hospital, the President of the Poor Law Board said

'Thank you for your enquiry re the system under which we conduct our workhouse and hospital. Up to about six months ago the whole institution was under the charge of the Master. We found that this mode of working resulted in constant friction between the two departments. As a result we decided to separate them, with the result that everything is now working most satisfactorily. Under our constitution the sole internal management of our Poor Law system is entrusted to the Vice President assisted by a House Committee of six appointed by the Poor Law Board."

Statistics for the late 1920s show that at the end of May 1928 there were 50 men and 44 women in the Hospital, 12 men and 17 women in the Asylum, and 63 children in the Children's Home, *'being (a total of) one more than the previous month and 6 more than May 1927'*. In January 1929 there were a total of 102 men, 70 women and 9 children in the establishments, but by August 1931 this had dropped to 75 men, 74 women and 6 children.

On a typical day at the Town Hospital in the inter-War period the Master and Matron would be up in time to start work when the Gate was opened at 7.00 a.m., and they would be on duty until 10.00 p.m. every night, and 10.30 p.m. on Saturdays. They had one half day off each week, and one full day once a fortnight.

The Master was responsible for admissions and discharges, burials, employment of all able-bodied inmates, their moral conduct and orderly behaviour. He had to visit the men's workshops and day-rooms every morning before 10 a.m., and make sure all fires and lights were out every night. He had to keep a daily record of all happenings and events, and had charge of the clothing and food stores and their issue. He was responsible for the requisition of all supplies, and he had to see that all inmates were fully employed and report on their work to each Board meeting. He also had the care of the key to the Dispensary and had to ensure every inmate was bathed on entry, and at least once a week thereafter.

Matron's duties were similar with regard to the female inmates. She also had to superintend the laundry, kitchen and sewing room. She had to ensure there were enough clothes made for the inmates, that laundry was washed and ironed on time, and that sufficient hot, properly cooked food was delivered to the wards and dining rooms every day. She was also responsible for the cleanliness of the establishment, and bathing the female inmates.

The female inmates were employed in the sewing room, laundry and kitchen. Women from outside the Hospital were also employed in the laundry, where they would scrub items in teak troughs with steam pipes underneath to keep the water hot.

The inmates were required to keep their dormitories and day rooms clean and tidy, and to clean other areas of the Hospital as required. When not doing other jobs the men would crack stone in the Labour Yard, on the other side of St Julian's Avenue. Some of them had small jobs, for example one was a scissor grinder and another mended shoes, but any money they earned went to the Hospital and they were given pocketmoney of about 1/- a week. For many years the Hospital hired out a sedan chair for people who wished to travel short distances around the Town, and the inmates carried this. They also made mats and other items which were sold.

The ambulance was kept at the Hospital and when this was required, the Second Master would go out with the driver and take an inmate to help him carry the other end of the stretcher.

From time to time the Hospital was isolated due to outbreaks of contagious diseases like smallpox, scarlet fever, influenza, and diphtheria. This did not always meet with the approval of the inmates, who wrote to the Board in 1904 complaining of the temporary closure due to an epidemic of diphtheria. The President paraded the signatories in front of everyone and *'severely admonished them for their impertinence and presumption in daring to question any action by the Management to deal with the affairs of the House'*. In 1921 there was another outbreak of the same disease. Cases were so numerous that the Sanatorium was full and two wards at the Infirmary were used as well.

The House Committee, together with the Master and Matron, tried hard to give the inmates as normal a life as possible within the constraints imposed on them. As well as special food on high days and holidays the poor were also given time off to celebrate events like Coronations and Royal Visits to the island. They took part in the Peace Celebrations in 1919, and both the Town Hospital and Asylum inmates had an annual picnic, on at least one occasion being taken to the Imperial Hotel at Pleinmont for a lobster tea at 1/8d per head.

They were taken for a drive and given tea afterwards to celebrate both Queen Victoria's Diamond Jubilee and Edward VIII's Coronation. When the Duke of Connaught came to unveil the War Memorial in 1905, the inmates were given a celebration tea followed by an entertainment under the direction of the Hospital chaplain, the Rev Clark.

They sat in the *'Cimitiere des Freres'* to see the King and Queen on their visit in 1921 and the Fruit Export Co. lent trolleys for them to stand on to see the Prince of Wales as he went up St Julians Avenue in 1936 on his way to open the Val des Terres. A former Board member left money in his will specifically for picnics for the inmates, and during the 1930s and 1940s a positive effort was made to provide entertainment, especially at Christmas time.

Disciplining the inmates was always difficult. Many were there because of drink problems, and by this time the only means of punishing them seemed to be putting them in the cells under the main hall for a period of time, on a diet of bread and water. Most inmates' idea of a day out was to save up their pocketmoney and go out and get absolutely drunk. On their return they would be put in the cells until they were sober again.

A few examples of behaviour which warranted punishment are - *'Thomas W having been granted a day's leave was brought in on the ambulance, drunk, at 10 p.m. Punishment - 3 month's leave stopped. Cara M. for insolence to Matron and Cook was sentenced to 24 hours in the cells on bread and water. Annie H. for striking Mrs Quartier and blackening her eye was brought before the House Committee, and then being defiant and noisy was locked up for the day.'*

The cells were condemned in 1902 as quite unsuitable, being dark, cold and insufficiently lit or ventilated. But they were still in use regularly for violent and abusive drunks as late as the 1950s.

During the Occupation

And then came the Second World War, and the occupation of Guernsey by the German Armed Forces.

All the sick and infirm from various institutions on the island, as well as the inmates of the Town Hospital, were brought together under one roof and for the next five years the Master and Matron performed a very difficult and extremely demanding job in an exemplary and most resourceful fashion. Their role in the care of the Island's sick and underprivileged during these years has been seriously undervalued.

In July 1940 the Poor Law Board was convened for a special meeting, to replace members who had left the island, as it had been pointed out by the Controlling Committee that *'it was desirable for the civic administration of the island to continue to function as in the past'*.

At the beginning of 1942 the Master requested some tea from the Essential Commodities Committee, but was sent 200 tins of pork and beans instead. There was a lack of money and fuel, and no uniforms so staff were given a uniform allowance. The President of the Poor Law Board said that, as authorised, he had amended the budget for 1942 but that his figures had not yet been accepted by the German authorities. The cost per day to keep an inmate in the Hospital at this time was 3/10d.

In September 1942 four members of staff were amongst those interned in Germany. The Controlling Committee instructed the Hospital to provide facilities for up to 250 people who were leaving the island, but in the end only six persons had to be accommodated. The States Supervisor issued an assurance that all members of staff deported would be reinstated in their positions, and that the time they were interned would count as service for pension and seniority purposes.

A report made by the German Commandant of the Channel Islands at this time (Oberst Knackfuss) acknowledged the cleanliness and general tidiness of the Hospital, and the President said he had been given to understand that this German had informed the Controlling Committee of his satisfaction with the manner in which the Institution was administered.

On the 25th and 26th March 1943 the Town Hospital was evacuated whilst the Germans had artillery practice. Some people went to St Stephen's Schoolroom and some to the Victoria Homes. The minutes noted that *'the Hospital would therefore be empty of all persons for certain hours on each day, an occurrence probably unprecedented in the whole history of the Institution'*.

Throughout the Occupation there was correspondence with those who were interned in Germany, and on 21 June 1944 a quantity of tinned goods which had been sent from Biberach was allocated to the Hospital. The amount received was approximately one third of the total, and a letter of thanks was sent to the Camp Captain expressing the Board's gratitude for these gifts.

In October 1944 there were 90 patients in the Infirmary, together with 10 staff, and an unknown number of inmates in the workhouse. Christmas Dinner that year consisted of meat stew and vegetables, with a jam duff baked by Warry's. By February 1945 there was no more bread, and Matron replaced it with bean and potato cake.

The Children's Home was moved to a new site at the Ivy Gates in March 1945, and Miss Harvey and the Girl Guides Association took it upon themselves to provide footwear and clothing for all the children, for which the authorities were very grateful.

The Canadian Red Cross had provided clothing and toys for the Channel Island evacuees in England during the War, and in August 1945 a representative visited the Hospital and asked for a list of the bedding and clothing required by the Hospital. The items were sent direct from Canada to Dr Collings. The following year Matron was given permission to attend the Victory Parade in London, but the police were refused permission to use the men's dining room for dancing practice, as being not practicable!

Not only did food shortages continue after the Occupation, but staff shortages were so acute that on more than one occasion the local branch of the St John Ambulance Association were asked if they could supply part time nurses to help in the Infirmary.

Numbers decline

The number of patients cared for in the Infirmary averaged between 80 and 100 in the years from 1950 to 1963, and appear to have been mostly the elderly chronically sick, whilst the number of inmates in the workhouse fell steadily. In July 1954 a recurring problem was identified with patients being transferred from the Princess Elizabeth Hospital who were usually covered in bedsores and often died within 48 hours.

There was further friction between the nursing and Workhouse sides of the establishment in 1955, apparently over the non-distribution of clean laundry, and in 1960 the Master and Matron, who were now called Superintendents, were moved out of their rooms as the Infirmary needed more room for patients. At this time the Board of Health agreed to support the building of a Nurses' Home within the precincts of the Hospital and agreed that there should be more beds for patients. They also asked for more co-operation between themselves and the 'Town Hospital Board'.

Matters seem to have come to a head in March 1963. A meeting was held at which the nursing staff said that there had been only five new admissions to the workhouse in the last year. Six inmates had been transferred to the infirmary and the remaining ten inmates should be absorbed into the infirmary as patients. It was now time for the Town Hospital to become solely a geriatric hospital. In answer to a question in the States, it was stated that in 1960, the States had appointed a committee of the Hospital Board, the Board of Health and the Insurance Authority to consider this matter, and that hopefully it would report soon.

In October of that year the Matron of the infirmary took over the care of the inmates, who she reported as being very dirty and in a low state of hygiene. Two were transferred to Jersey, leaving seven men and a woman who were subsequently cared for by the nurses. No difficulties were reported with this arrangement. The post of Superintendent ended as from 31 October, and effectively the Town Hospital ceased to exist as a workhouse from 1 November 1963. However it continued as a geriatric hospital for another 23 years.

Although the establishment had now become a geriatric hospital, discussions went on for a further seven years about which committee was actually in charge, the old Hospital Board, the Public Assistance Authority or the Board of Health.

Eventually some decision must have been made for in September 1969 there is a note in the minutes which says - *'While the question of the Board of Health taking over the St Peter Port Hospital had been mooted for some time the present recommendations had come quite unexpectedly'*.

The Board of Health takes over

The Hospital Board agreed to the proposal by 9 votes to 2, and in November 1969 the Board of Health finally took over the administration of the Town Hospital. In May 1970 they established a Geriatric Committee, one of whose responsibilities was the development of a co-ordinated geriatric service. The committee was also responsible for the administration of the Town Hospital, the K.E.VII Hospital and Les Cotils Nursing Home.

Throughout the 1970s there is a gradual process of change in the way the health services on the island are organised. In 1975 a memo noted that;

'When the new unit is completed at the K.E. VII Hospital, 50 fewer beds will be needed at St Peter Port Hospital'.

In 1977 following a Paper on the future of the geriatric services on the island it was stated that *'it would be helpful if an early decision could be taken as to whether or not St Peter Port Hospital was likely to be phased out over the next ten years or so'.*

Early in 1979 the States Engineer was asked to survey the Town Hospital with a view to its future use as a Police Station. The Board of Health told the Advisory and Finance Committee of its long term development proposals, and throughout that year discussions went ahead for an amalgamation of geriatric services at the K.E.VII Hospital and the eventual closure of the Town Hospital.

There was continuing political pressure to close the Town Hospital and in December 1983 letters began arriving asking for the Hospital building *'when it becomes vacant in two years time'.* A statement issued to the Press in September 1986 said that *'St Peter Port Hospital is to close in the autumn. The final date is not yet certain, and the patients will move when their condition has been assessed and accommodation has been found for them in the hospital which is most suited to their needs'.*

On 14 July 1987 the Chief Executive Officer of the Board of Health received a memo which bluntly stated- *'Will you please note that the St Peter Port Hospital has been completely cleared out and has been handed over to the Board of Administration, together with the keys'.*

So ended 245 years of care for the sick and underpriviledged at this establishment.

Food at the Town Hospital

The diet of inmates at the Hospital, though not necessarily what we would appreciate nowadays, was considered reasonable by the standards of the day. Breakfast was usually porridge, with thick slices of bread and butter and unlimited tea to drink.

Lunch was always a hot meal with vegetable soup or meat stew and vegetables, a suet pudding with fruit or jam in it, or rice or sago pudding, and tea to drink. If a dessert was not served at lunchtime it was often served at teatime, with bread and jam. The staff ate the same food, but it was often prepared differently, and they were also allowed extras like cheese and coffee.

It had always been recognised that some people needed a special diet for various reasons, and in 1901 these were recorded as *'Full, Half and Middle Diet'*. The extra items included mutton, fish, eggs, beef tea, alcohol and soda water. For example Mr R. had a full diet with extra beef tea, and Mr K. had extra mutton, milk, eggs and pudding. At the beginning of this century the average number of people fed at any one time varied between 125 and 130.

Food was rationed during the First World War, and became very scarce indeed during the Occupation. During 1917 all diets were revised to include more rice and less bread, and Matron was only allowed to continue giving bread to children under six when she explained that they could not digest the stews provided for them. Cook asked for and obtained a war bonus of 10/- a month whilst the special war diet was in force, as causing her more work.

High days and holidays were celebrated at the Hospital with hot cross buns on Good Friday, gâche on Midsummer Day, and roast beef and plum pudding on Christmas Day.

Clothing the poor

Clothes had always been provided for the poor, either to replace their existing clothing or as new clothes. As well as suits and dresses, people were given underclothes, coats, hats, boots and shoes and working clothes. The Hospital also bought material and made up the bedding it required. All staff were provided with uniforms, some items of which were made by the inmates, and the house badge was a pelican worked in worsted. However I can find no evidence of inmates wearing a uniform.

Tenders were usually invited for the supply of large amounts of material, and those bought were mostly the heavier, longer lasting textiles such as scotch linen, fustian, worsted and linsey. Flannelette was used to make nightclothes for the sick, as being more comfortable to wear, a material called *'ami des femmes'* was used for men's shirts, muslin was bought for the fever wards and white calico for shrouds. The clothes and bed linen were made by the female inmates and was a major part of the work they were expected to do.

Both adults and children could be provided with clothing when they left the Hospital. Emigrants usually received at least one full set of clothes, and two girls who went to Children's Homes in England were also provided with specialist clothing, probably a uniform of some kind.

The Lunatic Asylum

When the Town Hospital first opened in 1741 there was no public provision for the care of the mentally ill. At first they lived in the main house with everyone else but after a few years special rooms were built for them in the back yard. By 1849 their numbers had grown to such an extent that a special building was put up for them, which after the Second World War became what we now know as St Julians Hostel.

The Asylum had its own Master, Matron and nursing staff but was under the overall supervision of the Master of the Town Hospital. All its supplies were obtained through the Hospital and the Poor Law Board was responsible for employing its staff. The inmates had a sufficient although somewhat plain diet and were also usually included in any special events or celebrations that were organised for the inmates of the Town Hospital. The asylum inmates rose at 7.00 a.m. and were in bed by 10.00 p.m. Breakfast was at 7.30, lunch at 12.00 and tea at 6.00, and they spent their day 'in the grounds' although there is no record of exactly what they did. The doctor visited daily, usually in the afternoon.

In March 1916 electric light was installed at the Asylum, as being cheaper than gas, but a report in 1919 said that the building was no longer considered satisfactory for the treatment of the insane. However as the States had agreed some fourteen years earlier to build an asylum for the whole island it was decided that it was not worth while upgrading it.

By the end of the First World War the men had been moved to the Country (Castel) Hospital. A note of the diagnoses for the women in the Town Asylum in 1934 includes endocrine imbalance, premature senility, hyperthyroidism, anaemia, malnutrition, cardiac aesthenia and chronic dyspepsia. A former resident of the Hospital said that before a person was sent to the Asylum they had to be certified by two doctors, and they were sometimes at the Hospital for weeks. They often made a great deal of noise and were sometimes put in a straightjacket to stop them harming themselves.

The Childrens Home

The Town Hospital had always cared for orphans and the children of the poor. In 1746 there is a record of a Mary Papplestone, pauper child, being returned to her relatives in London, and it was also appreciated that babies and young children should have their own living and sleeping areas.

In 1900 the building on the site of what is now States Housing flats was used as the Children's Home, supervised by the Matron of the Town Hospital. The children in the Home were either illegitimate children whose mothers could not look after them, or orphans. Young girls would be admitted pregnant to the Hospital, work until they had their baby, and then be found a job and go back to work and the baby was placed in the Children's Home.

The children were given a similar diet to the adults although they had more milk. All their clothes were provided, including hats, shoes, and accessories like umbrellas. The authorities tried to be as sympathetic as possible, and in 1918 Miss Le Noury was asked not to make more than three dresses of the same pattern for the girls. The children were educated at parish expense, and later apprenticed into various jobs. They also had the opportunity to emigrate if they wished. There was a continuing problem with the temporary care of boys who were on their way to reformatories, later known as Borstal, and to industrial schools in England and attempts were made to employ these boys whilst they were awaiting transfer.

In the 1930s the Home was moved to Greenfields but towards the end of the Occupation it moved to a house at the Ivy Gates and the Hospital Matron was again asked to supervise it. By 1950 the Home had moved back to Greenfields. It was administered by the Children Board and all connection with the Town Hospital severed.

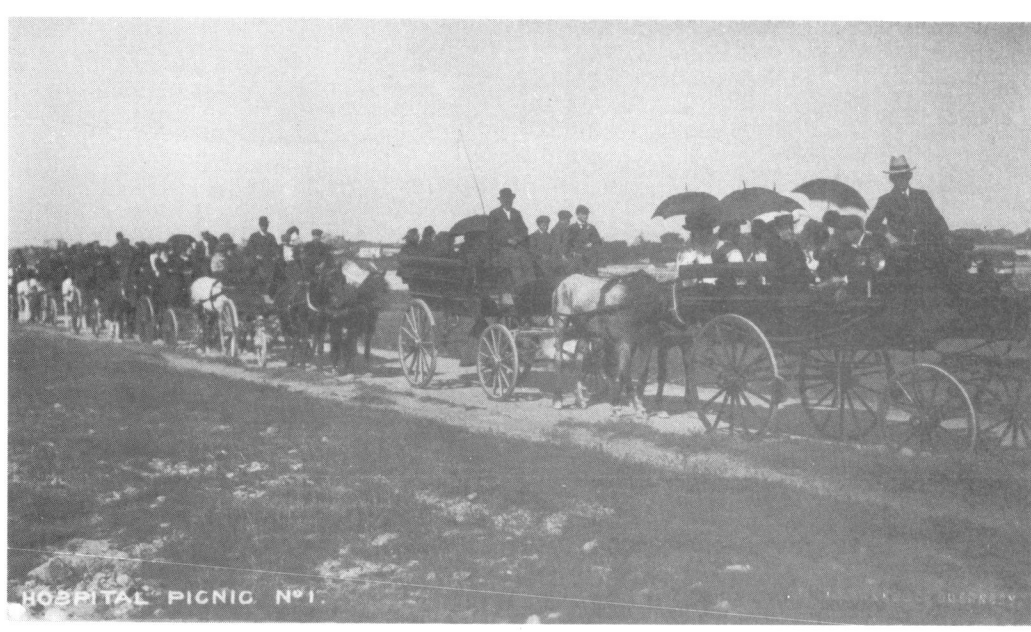

Town Hospital Picnic and Inmates at the Imperial Hotel, Pleinmont 1911

'*The House Committee* (of the Town Hospital) *together with the Master and Matron tried to give the inmates as normal a life as possible within the constraints imposed on them .... both the Town Hospital and the Asylum inmates had an annual picnic, on at least one occasion being taken to the Imperial Hotel at Pleinmont for lobster tea at 1/8d'*. (Chapter Three)

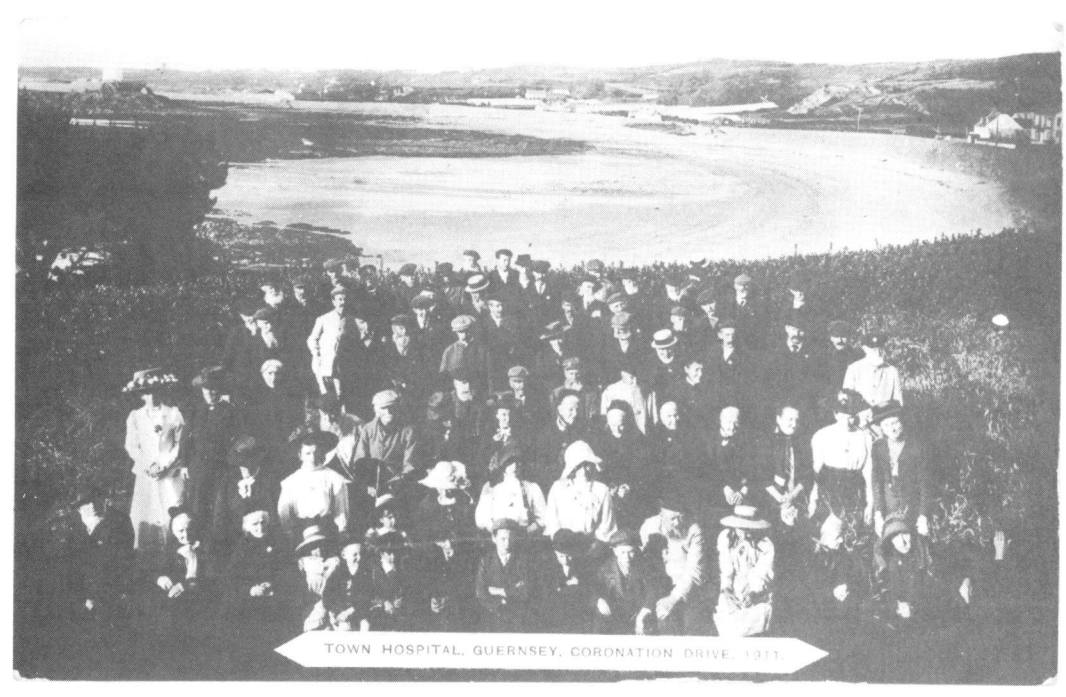

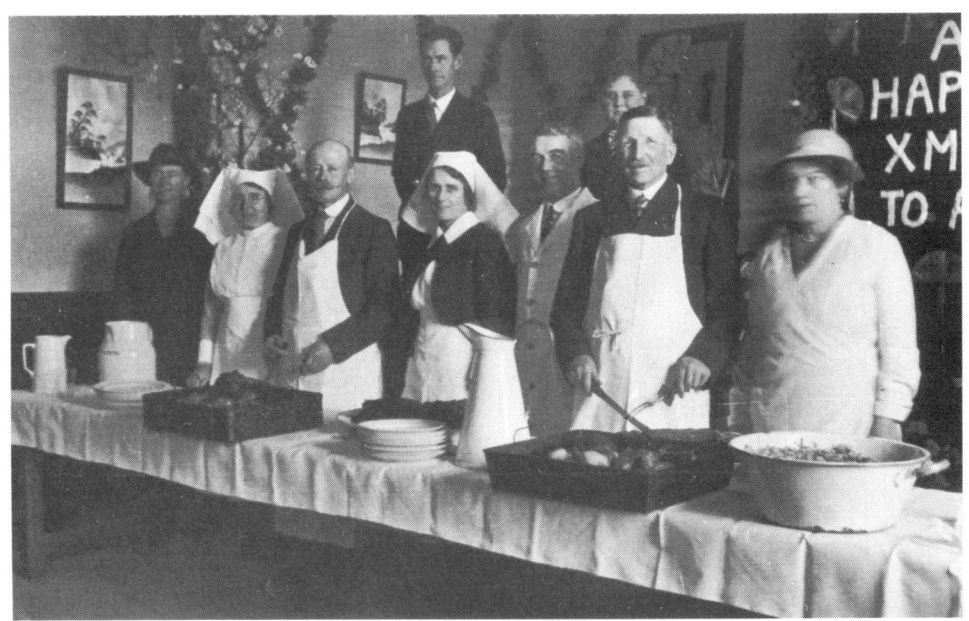

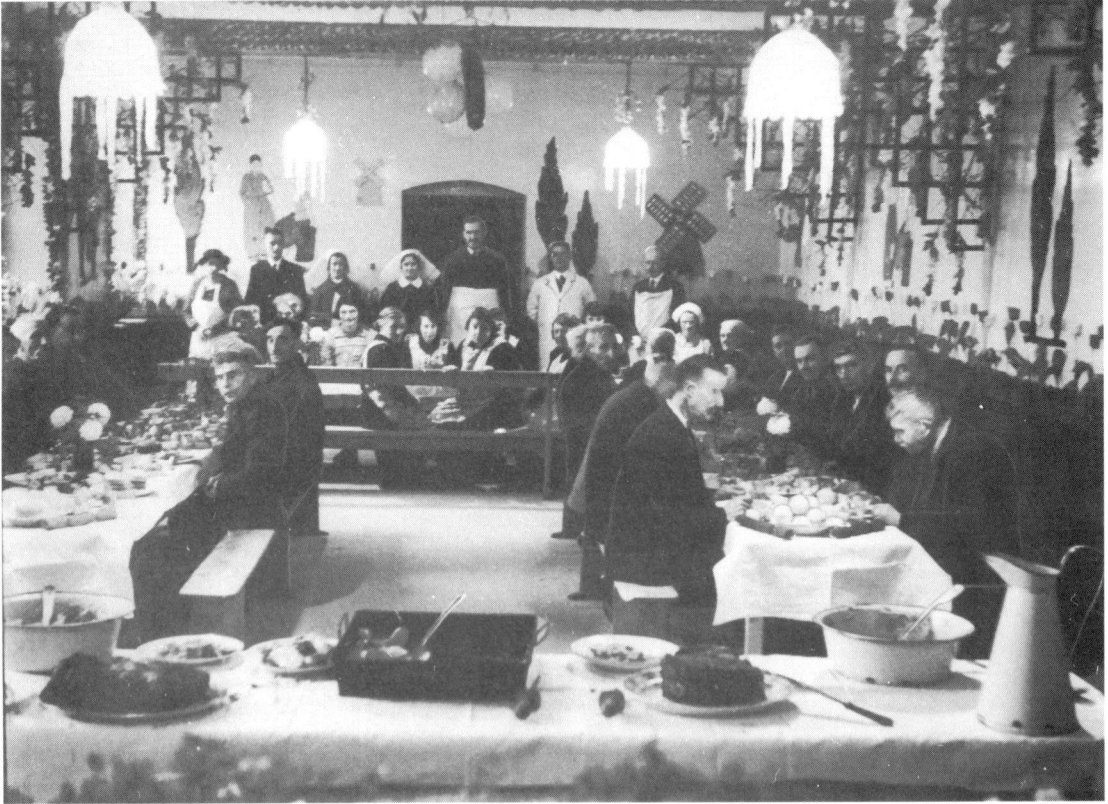

At the Town Hospital - Christmas Day 1938

'High days and holidays were celebrated at the Hospital with hot cross buns on Good Friday, gâche on Midsummer's Day, and roast beef and plum pudding on Christmas Day'.

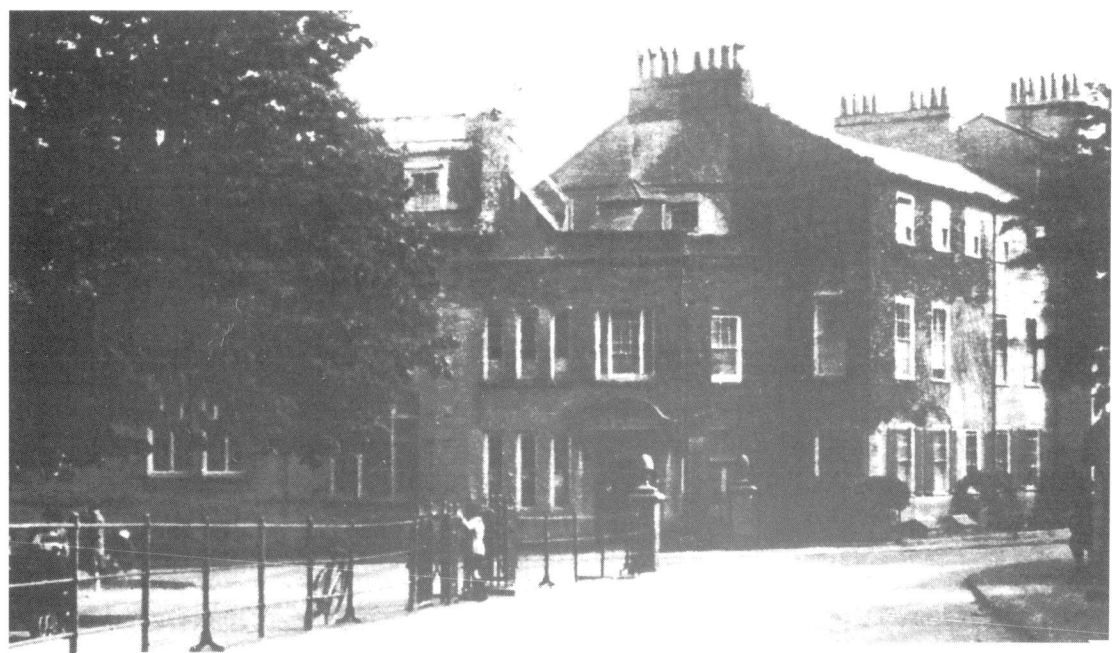

The Victoria Cottage Hospital at its second site in Park House, Cambridge Park (now the Duke of Richmond Hotel) around 1891. This was followed by the move to the former 'St John's Industrial Girls Home' (now Amherst) in 1898. (Chapter Four)

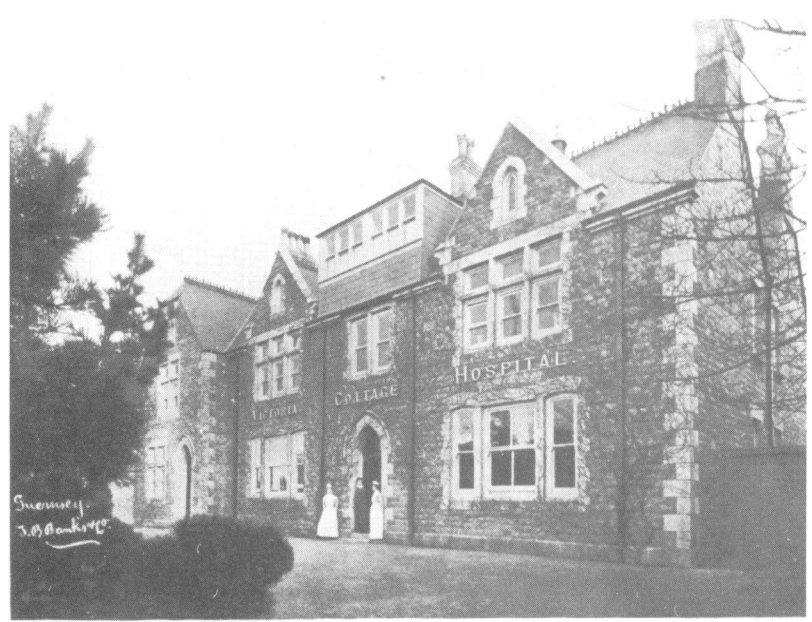

THE VICTORIA COTTAGE HOSPITAL, GUERNSEY.

T. B. Banks & Co., Central Library, Guernsey

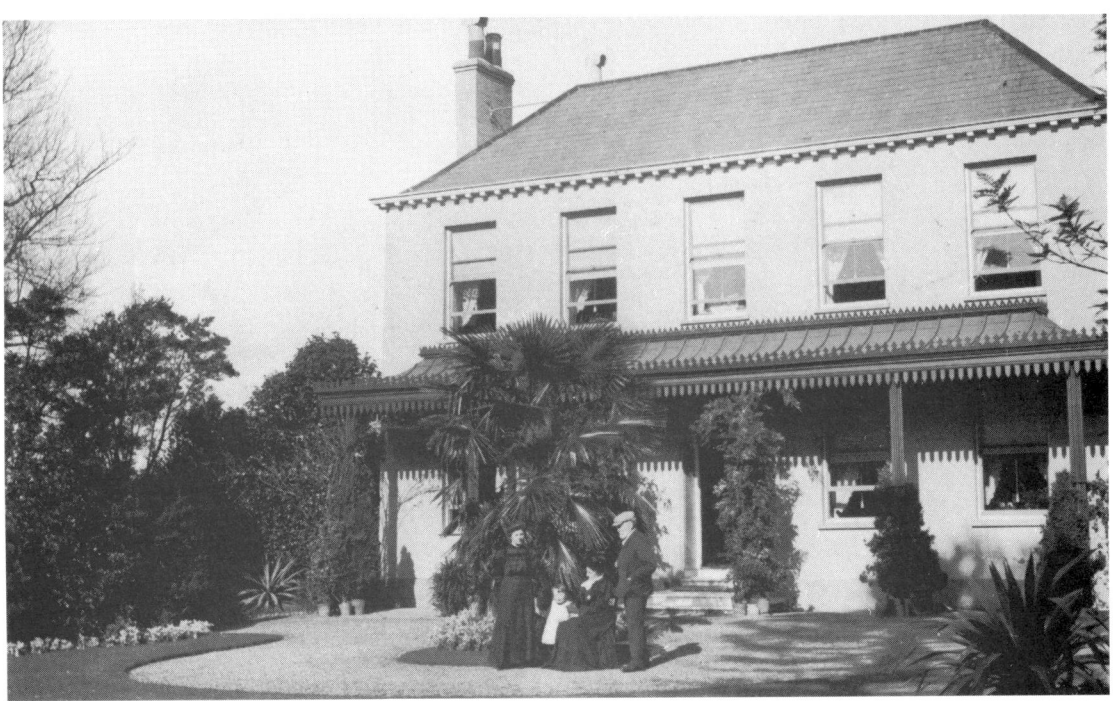
Valnord House around 1900 when still a private residence (Chapter Six)

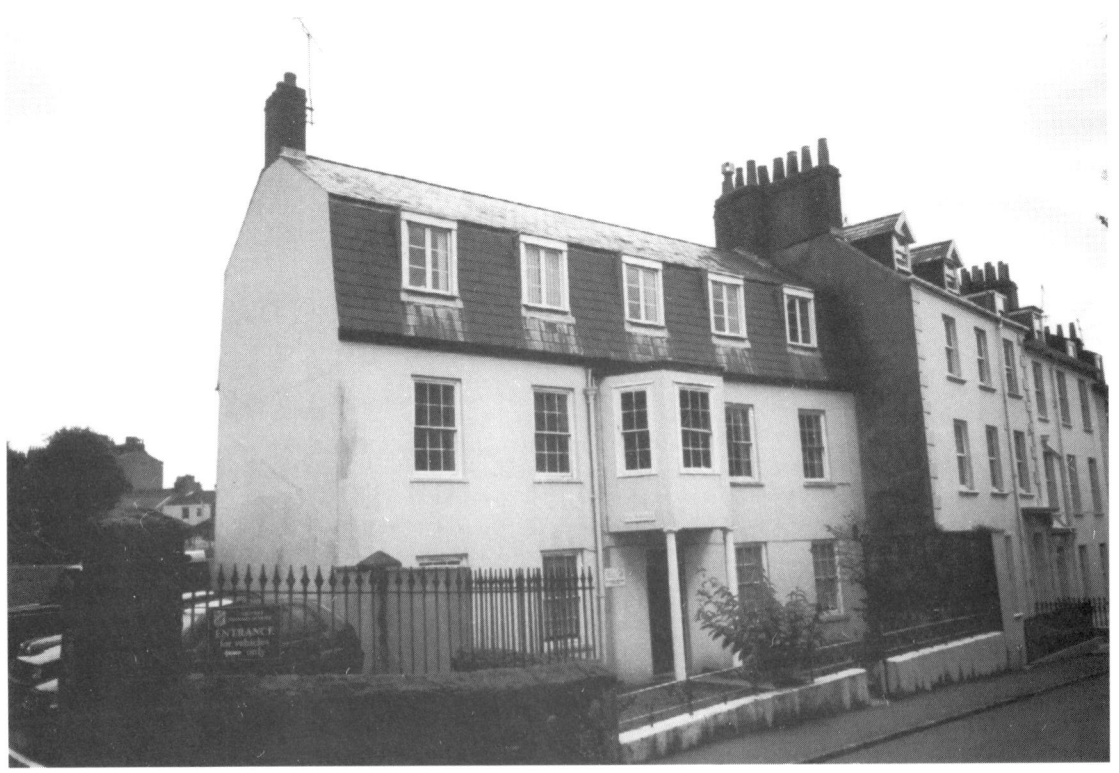
Floraville as it is today (Chapter Six)

Chapter Four

The Victoria Cottage Hospital (Amherst)

W T Gallienne

The 'respectable poor' were reluctant to seek admission to both the Town and Country Hospitals because of the perceived stigma of their 'Poor Law' origins. Dr E Laurie Robinson had the vision to propose a 'Guernsey Cottage Hospital' and the drive and determination to seek the funds needed to turn this vision into reality. The Victoria Hospital was in turn, Cottage Hospital, hospital for British Troops during World War One and German Troops during World War Two, and finally a maternity home before the last patients left in March 1980.

The need for a Cottage Hospital

The principal reason for the establishment of a 'Cottage Hospital'; was the lack of good nursing facilities. Prior to 1887 there were only two hospitals, both administered by the Poor Law Board. They were the St Peter Port Hospital which became known as the Town Hospital, and the Country Hospital which later became the Castel Hospital. Professional nursing was almost non existent; the nursing staff generally being untrained. Although the doctors were usually well trained, the facilities they had to work in were mostly basic, with very little surgical equipment. Doctors chosen by the hospitals were the only ones allowed to practice within that institution, local practitioners found it difficult to get someone admitted, they had to deal with each in the patient's home, with friends and family doing the nursing. Although these charity hospitals were better than nothing. The 'respectable poor' often felt disgraced if they had to be admitted into them.

At the beginning of 1887 a *'St Peter Port Nursing Corps'* was formed by Dr E. Laurie Robinson using ladies who had 'First Aid' and 'Nursing' Certificates in the St John's Ambulance Association. After further training they were sent out to help nurse the sick in their own homes. Their success brought the desire for a permanent place where patients could be looked after. Better care by the doctors using up to date equipment and good nursing was envisaged.

A 'Guernsey Cottage Hospital' is proposed

Doctor Robinson in a course of lectures to 90 nursing students in the autumn of 1887 told them of his idea to establish a 'Cottage Hospital' in Guernsey. He asked them to see how much they could raise in subscriptions or donations toward the project. At the end of the year £140 in annual subscriptions and £30 in donations were pledged. With this encouragement he called a meeting with the medical practitioners. He outlined his plan to them and soon found their support and approval. An advertisement appeared in 'The Star' of 14th January 1888 proposing a cottage hospital as follows;

'A movement is a foot to establish an Institution of this character, and a public meeting is announced to be held at 3 o'clock under the presidency of Sir Edgar MacCulloch in the room at the Young Mens Christian Association, in order to bring the subject more prominently before the public. All who are interested in the movement are invited to be present'.

So on 19th January 1888 at 3 pm a meeting took place at the YMCA room in the States Arcade for the subscribers and the general public under the chairmanship of the Bailiff, Sir Edgar MacCulloch. The following report appeared in 'The Star':

'Guernsey Cottage Hospital'

'A meeting of the subscribers and supporters of the above scheme held in the YMCA room yesterday afternoon, under the presidency of Sir Edgar MacCulloch, Bailiff'.

'The Bailiff in opening the proceedings, said that all present had felt for some time past the need of a Hospital, such as it was proposed to establish, an Institution where the respectable poor could be taken where they would not mix with bad characters to be found in the General Hospitals. With Guernseymen the word hospital was almost inseparably connected with disgrace and crime, the Poor House in fact, but in the Cottage Hospital stringent rules would be adopted to keep out all impure characters. Voluntary subscriptions would be needed to float the scheme. He called on Dr Robinson to unfold the scheme to the meeting'.

'Dr Robinson said he was glad to see so many present, the establishment of a branch of the St John's Ambulance Association had considerable influence in carrying out his dream of a Cottage Hospital in Guernsey. There were some 250 of these hospitals in England, the first being at Cranley in Surrey. At the present time there was not a single hospital bed supported by voluntary contributions in Guernsey. In our flourishing community the well-to-do ought to feel responsibility towards the poor. Although there are General Hospitals in the island, they are so mixed up with the work-house that the respectable poor have great objection to go there on account of the disgrace. There should he some place for the decent poor to go in case of illness'.

'He went on to say that to make a hospital work well, the medical officers should be ex officio members of the Board, as in all voluntary hospitals in England, whereas in the Poor Houses they are merely paid officers with very little voice in the management'.

'Finance was the chief question, not one of the Cottage Hospitals was endowed, there expenses being met in five ways: annual subscriptions, donations, Hospital Sunday, patient's payments and interest on funded property. The greatest proportion of this, about 54% comes from annual subscriptions. It would he impossible to start with a new building, but the idea is to rent a suitable house'.

'It was proposed to commence with four beds. This did not sound very much, but we must go slowly at first. The cost was estimated in this manner, the expenses including the rent, housekeeping and salaries of nurses and servants, divided by the amount of the average number of beds occupied during the year was believed to be £60 per annum for each bed, so for four beds the total cost would be £240. I have been asked "Will it pay?" My reply being, financially no, but by relieving the respectable poor and bringing credit to the island, yes. No infectious or incurable diseases would be admitted. All medical men in the island have agreed to support the hospital, so that every patient would be attended by their own doctor. The nursing at first would be carried out by the Ladies of the St Peter Port Nursing Corps, under a trained matron. The management would be in the hands of all the medical officers and lay members elected by the subscribers. There would also be a sub committee, on which the speaker and Dr Collings had been chosen to represent the medical staff. A Ladies' Committee would be appointed to help in the housekeeping, etc. Each patient would be allowed a visit by his own Minister, of whatever creed'.

'At present we have only enough money to work three beds. But there was a possibility of 'Memorial Beds'. Such beds would have a brass plate over them with any name selected by the donors on them. The cost to the donor would be about £20. The money would about pay for bed, bedding and necessary furniture. The Rev. G E Lee thought the scheme would be a success as it had been taken up warmly by the medical men. The idea of 'Memorial Beds' was good. Thomas Guille Esq, [famous for the Guille Alles Library] thought the idea was a good one, but thought that the institution should not be called a hospital as there was such a prejudice against all such in the island. Dr Robinson said "Let us stick to the name 'hospital' and teach the people here what such a name really means". A vote of thanks was given to the Bailiff for presiding. In reply he said he had been quite ignorant of the subject, but the clear and lucid explanation of Dr Robinson had thoroughly enlightened him. He agreed with Mr Guille, he thought the word 'hospital' was distasteful to the respectable poor. Thomas Guille proposed and Rev Lee seconded the vote of thanks to Dr Robinson'.

A second meeting was held on 2nd February 1888 to appoint a committee. Rev F E Lowe chaired the meeting in the absence of the Bailiff. It was well attended with a large number of ladies present. It was announced that the Bailiff had consented to become President of the Hospital. Col Durand was unanimously elected Hon Secretary, and Sausmarez Le Cocq was elected Hon Treasurer. The rest of the committee consisted of the medical officers and Messrs The Rev G E Lee, Julius Carey, General Le Cocq, Major Dutton, R De Lisle, Rev F E Lowe, Thomas Guille, Rev Martin P F Carey, Dr M MacCulloch, Col Collings and F M Allès. The Ladies Committee consisted of Mrs Nicholls, Mrs Frank Carey, Mrs Dutton, Miss Mary Collings, Mrs John E Collings, Miss Mollett and Mrs Carey.

The same meeting was told that the subscription list amounted to £190. Two memorial beds had been promised, one by the Misses Woolcombe and one by Mrs W Bainbridge in memory of her son.

After some discussion on the name of the establishment, it was decided to leave the naming of the institution to the General Committee.

Early days of the new hospital

On 1st May, the first Hospital was opened. There had been some difficulty in finding suitable premises, as no one seemed to want their house to become a hospital, but eventually 2 St George's Place, Candie Road was rented. After some reorganisation of the house, six beds were able to be accommodated within it. Two beds were located downstairs for men, three beds upstairs for women, and one bed was provided for operation cases, and a room used as an operating theatre. Miss Tourtel from Alderney was appointed the first Matron. She helped the hospital financially by refusing to accept any kind of salary for the first year.

The Bailiff performed the opening ceremony by turning the key and opening the door. The Matron and several of the nurses were the first to enter and shortly behind them the general public. A short service of dedication was offered by Rev Lee at the entrance to the female ward.

At the first Annual General Meeting on 26th January 1889, the Committee expressed their conviction that the Hospital's great popularity had already proved its benefit to the island. Wards were constantly full, and in fact there was a waiting list. A variety of patients were accepted, the majority were of the grade of people intended. Just eight months after the opening of the Hospital, thirty two patients had been admitted, nineteen females, and thirteen males, which would average forty eight in one year. There had been just one death, twelve operations had been performed, some serious, but all were successful. It was satisfactory to note that the expenses of the hospital were less than any other Cottage Hospital of its size in England.

On account of ill health Miss Tourtel resigned in February 1890 after a short but dedicated service. The Committee decided that it would not be the appropriate thing to use the Hospital funds to present her with a parting gift, especially since she had refused her first year's salary. It was therefore agreed that each member of the Committee would donate not less than ten shillings. They must have been very generous for she was later presented with a Queen Anne silver tea-service. Her post was taken by Miss Gadsby of the London Hospital.

In 1890 an extension to 2 St George's Place was considered, by taking over the house next door, but the scheme fell through. However an advantageous loan of £700 was raised in December which made it possible to purchase Park House, Cambridge Park, now the Richmond Hotel, which was described as *'very commodious'* and would supply all present needs. A vote of thanks was made to the Ladies' Committee by Dr Robinson who said that when the suggestion was first made some one had said *"Why talk about a Ladies Committee they will spoil it all? All he wished to say was if it had not been for them, the Hospital would not have succeeded"*. After refurbishment, the new Hospital was opened by the Bailiff on 21st April 1891. The following year the Committee deemed advisable, because of the increased costs of a larger building to open a private ward for a better (paying) class of patient. Seven people availed themselves of this facility in the first year.

Fund raising was always a problem, although there were many regular benefactors. Collections were made in churches and chapels in the island. In 1894 £63 5s 11d was raised in this way, although there were still many prejudices to be overcome. Dr Robinson said that he had heard it stated that *"all patients entering the hospital died there, but he was prepared to prove them wrong. Over a three year period the average deaths had been 4.8%, 1% less than any other Country Hospital"*. This he said spoke volumes for the treatment received at the Hospital. The Matron of St Thomas' Hospital in London on a visit had expressed in the highest terms the good general arrangement of the Hospital.

On 15th February 1897 a special meeting was called to consider an offer made in a letter written by William Carey, Secretary to the Guernsey Industrial Home for Girls, Amherst. In it, he wrote that in consequence of a decision to close the Home, it had been resolved to offer the premises to the Victoria Cottage Hospital, for its purposes. To supplement the offer they promised £100 from the Home Fund for a period of five years, toward the expenses of the Hospital. They were also prepared to spend some sums of money, within reason, toward the conversion of the building. The generous offer was accepted unanimously.

That the offer came to be made in the first place, was due to the terms upon which the Industrial Home had been established. Nicholas Carey in his youth had left Guernsey and resided in many parts of the world before finally settling back in the island in 1870, at the age of about 64. His interests then turned to good works. He was involved in the Society for the Prevention of Cruelty to Animals and was the founder of the St John's Girls Industrial Home, which later became the Guernsey Industrial Home for Girls. On his death he left part of his fortune to the Home and part to Miss Henrietta Corbin, sister to Dr M A B Corbin. A codicil to his Will stated in effect that if the Home should fail in the purpose for which it had been founded, then it would be for the Committee to hand it over to some other suitable institution of their choice.

The move to Amherst

Just over a year later, after extensive work had been undertaken to convert the building into a hospital, and with a gathering of about one hundred patrons, despite the high wind and showers, the Hospital was opened by the Lieutenant Governor, General Stevenson. Wards were now large, unlike the previous hospitals which had smaller rooms. In each ward hung a portrait of the person after whom the ward had been named. Each iron bed was covered in a red flannel counterpane, and each bed named by the donor, for example Willie, Bankipore, Dobrèe, etc. The operating theatre had been fitted out with all the latest improvements.

In 1903 a further improvement was made. A Rontgen X-ray machine had been installed which would be useful to determine fractures and the whereabouts of metal and bullets in the body. Moreover the rays were considered to be useful for the cure of Lupus and other skin diseases.

Dr Robinson in his report to the annual general meeting in 1906 said that the example of the Victoria Cottage Hospital had led to improvements in the other establishments in the island. Mr Peter Carey, Vice President of the Poor Law Board of St Peter Port had visited and had *'learnt a few wrinkles'*. Everyone knew the Town Hospital was not what it had been, but there was still room for improvement in the Country Hospital.

By 1908 the Hospital had over twenty five beds available, 2,732 patients had been received, one hundred and twenty seven deaths had occurred, or about 4%. There had been nine hundred and thirty one operations undertaken, with thirty five deaths, about $3^1/_2$%. Considering all sorts of cases were received these figures were thought to be good.

Generally all the matrons had been very good and highly thought of by the Committee, that is except for Miss Maclagan who resigned on 28th April 1909, taking with her the whole of the nursing staff, apparently over a report made to the Committee about the running of the Hospital and the wastefulness that went on. In June 1909 one hundred and twenty applications were received for the post of matron. Miss Edith Bond was finally chosen. Her duties commenced on 1st August with a complete new nursing staff.

With the Sanatorium having opened in 1902, and the Victoria Cottage Hospital now fully established, Dr Robinson observed that Guernsey could be proud from a medical point of view - *"Jersey medical men were green with envy as they had nothing like it"*.

During the First World War after an inspection by officials of the War Office, the Victoria Cottage Hospital was recognised as a Class A Hospital. Dr Robinson was appointed Special Surgeon to the Forces in Guernsey and Alderney, and many hundreds of Servicemen were treated there during the War.

At the March meeting of 1918, consideration was given to whether the name Cottage should be dropped, as it was thought that the hospital had now outgrown such a description. In April approval for the name change was agreed, and so it became known as The Victoria Hospital.

Various changes took place over the years, one of the biggest being the departure of Dr Robinson from the medical staff of the Hospital in 1924, although he continued to be a member of the Committee. At a meeting on 7th May 1925, the Hon Treasurer stated that payments had fallen, primarily because the Hospital had been partially closed owing to lack of nursing staff. This seems to have instigated a series of alterations. On 1st May 1926 the Hospital closed to modernise the nursing quarters, renew the piping and replace the fire escape. Two open air wards were opened, for men and women respectively, and a new x-ray plant was installed. The Hospital re-opened on 10th September 1926.

Plans for expansion

It was becoming clear by 1928 that the Committee would have to provide additional accommodation, as the popularity of the Hospital was growing. Fund raising was always a problem, and from the beginning money was found by subscriptions, rents, gifts, etc and a 'Pound Day' where people would give a pound or more, or goods to that value, toward upkeep. Open days were organised where visitors were allowed to wander freely over the Hospital. A report in the Star Newspaper gave a description of what took place on the day. Visitors even peeped into the nurses' bedrooms, and made a thorough inspection of the operating theatre (which cannot have been such an awesome place to these casual visitors as it undoubtedly was to the patients). Time was spent watching Mr T W Rylatt, the Radiologist pointing out the interesting features of the many x-ray negatives and photographs.

Notwithstanding its early sophistication, by the 1930's it was recognised that the Hospital needed to be brought into line with current medical standards. A joint meeting held on 25th January 1934 to hear a report that had been commissioned in September of the previous year on the building of a new hospital. Mr Orde, the Director of the Central Bureau of Hospital Information, and the Honorary Secretary of The British Hospital Association, made the following four points.

1. A building for about sixty beds was required.

2. There was enough space on the site to extend.

3. There was need for considerable improvement.

4. An expert hospital architect should be asked to make a report on how the present building could be made into an adequate hospital.

Little more took place regarding building a new hospital, except that the Hospital was closed for a month in July of the following year for further alterations to take place. An indication of how numbers of patients had grown over the last fifty years came at a meeting in June 1935 when the following figures were given:

1895	=	89
1905	=	230
1915	=	274
1925	=	348
1935	=	560

In November 1935 it was announced that a ward was to be named after Dr Robinson.

Miss Daisie Mignot of the Lady Ozanne Maternity Home (which had opened in 1922) wrote to the Committee on 5th June 1936 to arrange a meeting to discuss a union between the Maternity Home and the Victoria Hospital. Some co-operation did take place, but they were never fully amalgamated.

Because of the various potential legal liabilities facing the Trustees, it was thought by the Committee that incorporation was necessary and a requete was presented to the States. Incorporation duly took place on 22nd July 1936.

An Extraordinary Meeting was held on 28th December 1938 to discuss a letter received from the Island Hospital Committee, asking if the Victoria Hospital Incorporated would be willing to combine with the proposed new Island Hospital. This idea found favour with the Committee and various suggestions were made, but no decision taken. Instead a letter was sent to the Island Hospital Committee asking them to elaborate. The President of the Committee D A Aubert replied on 11th January 1939 detailing the scheme as it would be presented to the States. It recommended that an Island Hospital be erected by the States, and that the Victoria Hospital Corporation would become the tenants, and manage the Island Hospital. The existing buildings would be taken over by the States at an agreed valuation, bringing the whole hospital under one ownership. A detailed change in the rules to enable the Committee to be increased to 30 was also produced. The Corporation would also have to undertake to accept liability for accommodating all sick poor requiring medical and surgical treatment. They would also be responsible for the management of a suggested Contributory Scheme. Unfortunate events were about to delay any such change of ownership.

Dr Robinson died in March 1939 just more than a year before the Hospital was taken over by the German Occupying Forces. It saved him the distress of having to see all his efforts ruined by the war. On 24th June 1940 a letter was received from Dr Symons, the Medical Officer of Health, informing the Committee that until further notice the Victoria Hospital Corporation was in abeyance, and that all patients would be evacuated to the Country Hospital along with all stores, etc. It was five long years before the States and the Corporation would need to report on the future of the Victoria Hospital.

Post war change

After the war the Corporation placed a claim for war damage with the Channel Islands' (Property) Rehabilitation Scheme which had been announced in August 1945. The assessors stated that the Hospital had been occupied by the Germans and although there was considerable wear and tear as a result, the general condition was fair. They assessed the minimum figure needed to re-establish the Hospital to be £450 for the building itself, £150 for the nurses' home and £3,584 for equipment. The Corporation had very few funds left, the system of collecting through subscriptions had lapsed over the five years of Occupation, and to establish it again would be virtually impossible.

In September Dr Symons explained the problem about re-opening the Hospital. The cost of repairs to the damage caused by the Germans would make it inadvisable. He suggested handing the Hospital over to the Lady Ozanne Maternity Home. A Sub-Committee was set up in December to report back to the Corporation. After considering that report it was decided to offer the Victoria Hospital building to the States at a fair valuation.

Dr Symons told the Board of Health Committee that the Victoria Hospital Corporation had decided to sell the buildings and land, and they were giving the first option to the States to purchase. Members of the Board wondered if the Corporation would agree to giving the buildings and land as a free gift, in view of the financial position the States found itself in, and the fact that it would remain a hospital.

A statement made by Mr S W Milburn FRIBA, who had been retained by the States to make reports on the hospitals, considered the conversion of the Hospital into a maternity home and ante-natal clinic to be a very good idea. It was, he said, a fine building designed for what was required. To ascertain what would be required in the way of structural alterations to convert the building to a maternity centre, Dr A O Bisson and Dr W B Fox, accompanied by the States Engineer, visited the Victoria Hospital in August 1946. Dr Fox thought the hospital would be suitable, but envisaged a shortage of rooms for private patients. One ward would be lost to accommodate the babies, and there could be four private wards. The total beds available would be thirty two, but no room was available to accommodate an anti natal clinic. A valuation of the property was made for the Corporation by Mr Hunkin at £11,642, and by Mr Lainé the States Engineer at £10,932. The Committee voted to ask for the lower figure from the States. On 11th December 1946 the States agreed to buy the Victoria Hospital from the Corporation for the sum asked for, and a further sum of £3,900 was voted to refurbish the Hospital and to turn it into the Island Maternity Hospital.

With the war having just finished, materials were sometimes hard to acquire, and therefore delays were inevitable. To exacerbate things further, dry rot was found in the joists, which cost an additional £3,500 to rectify. At the end of the conversion the Board of Health had spent approximately £11,000 in total, well over the £3,900 voted initially by the States. For nearly three decades most island births were to take place at the refurbished premises.

By the 1970's pressures on the health services in the island were being felt. Various reviews were made to try and make better use of the buildings and the trained staff overseen by the Board of Health. It was considered a benefit to both mothers and babies if the maternity services were transferred to the Princess Elizabeth Hospital. This would also make best use of the trained staff. An announcement was made in 1973 that from 18th June all maternity patients would go direct to the Princess Elizabeth Hospital. Patients would be allowed to go home after two or three days, but if further post-natal care was needed then they would be transferred to the Amherst Hospital for convalescence.

The knell for the Hospital came in March 1980, when the willingness of the Board of Health to release the Amherst Hospital for use as a temporary Police Station, was confirmed, provided that alternative accommodation could be found for the Board of Health staff.

A sum of £78,000 was voted by the States for the building's conversion. With that vote, its long association with health and care in the community came to an end. It would be interesting to have Dr Robinson's views on the growth of healthcare in the island since those small beginnings in 1887, which he had so enthusiastically promoted.

Main sources

Short History of The Victoria Hospital by E Laurie Robinson (Priaulx Library)
Minute Book of The Victoria Hospital (Priaulx Library)
Minutes Books of the Board of Health (Island Archive Service)
States Billets D'Etat (Island Archive Service)
Star and Guernsey Evening Press (Priaulx Library)

Chapter Five

Mental Health Services

Adrian Gaggs

The care of the mentally unwell was long linked with the care of other indigents. Although the need for improved provision of care was identified in the 1930s, it was not until after World War Two that a specialist psychiatric service began to develop. The Castel Hospital was central to the care of the mentally ill throughout this period, until the concepts of 'community care' began to be accepted in the 1970s.

Origins of mental health care in Guernsey

The care of the mentally unwell in Guernsey was for many years closely linked with the care of the poor and those unable to work through physical incapacity.

Prior to the States taking over the relief and care of the poor and needy, this responsibility belonged to the ecclesiastical side of Parish administration. The *'Procureur des Pauvres'* was the relief officer, assisted by four *'Collecteurs des Pauvres'*, elected by the ratepayers of that parish. Before the Reformation, the poor, sick and elderly, and those with mental infirmities were dependent on the generosity of the charitably minded.

During Queen Elizabeth I's reign and with the onset of Calvinist Presbyterianism there were the beginnings of Parish relief. In the Sixteenth Century the Churchwardens were called, for example, *'Les Collecteurs du Tresor de l'eglise de St Pierre Port'* and looked after the poor. In 1611 the cost of poor relief was charged on the rates. In 1725 the levying of poor rates was general in all the parishes and called *'La Taxe des Pauvres'*. The *'Collecteurs des Pauvres'*, (four to each Parish), collected this and handed in the proceeds to the Churchwardens *(Les Tresoriers)*. In 1720 the *'Procureur des Pauvres'*, a parochial officer, relieved the Churchwardens of their poor relief duties.

The poor were sub-divided into three categories - (1) ordinary native residents, (2) stranger poor - non-natives, usually given enough money for them to be repatriated, and (3) 'Les Pauvres Honteux' - these were the elderly, the sick, widows, spinsters and men unable to work. They were given flour at Whitsun, Michaelmas and Christmas from a special fund.

In 1741 the Town Hospital was founded by the ratepayers of St Peter Port and ten years later seven of the country parishes banded together to provide a similar establishment - the Country Hospital in the Castel for the aged and infirm. In 1798 St Peter-in-the-Wood joined in with the country parishes in funding the Country Hospital and in 1826 the Forest also joined in its funding.

The term 'hospital' was used for the following categories of people - (1) the poor and destitute, (2) as a shelter for drunks and socially inadequate people as an alternative to prison, (3) the mentally ill, mentally handicapped and elderly who could not be looked after at home, and (4) orphans and children abandoned by their parents.

The beginnings of centralised health care

A century later, in 1899 came the appointment of a Medical Officer of Health and the appointment of the Board of Health as described in Chapter One. The Board of Health was not responsible for the hospitals, but only had an advisory role to the Douzaines in protecting the public health.

In 1902 the Kind Edward VII Sanatorium for Infectious Diseases was established as an open-air treatment for tuberculosis, becoming the first hospital run by the Board of Health.

As far back as 1903, the States Asylum Committee had reported that *'the existing asylums are altogether unsuited for the proper treatment of mental diseases'*. Various ideas and plans were considered, but nothing definite was decided and the Great War stopped any further progress in this direction.

A document entitled *"Hôpital de la Campagne, Ordinance et Reglement"* dated 1916 confirms that the Country hospital was still being used for the poor, the infirm, children and "lunatics" at that date. It gives very precise regulations for the "inmates". For example, Article 16 states - *'All the inmates, except the sick, during the months of November, December, January and February, shall arise at 6.30am, during the months from March to October inclusive, at 5.30am. They shall retire at 7.30pm from November to February inclusive and at 8.30pm from March to October inclusive; while understood that in cases of necessity the Masters and Mistresses shall be allowed keep up such as they may think fit, to assist them out of the aforementioned hours'*.

Article 17 required, *'All the inmates, except the sick and the infirm, shall assemble when the bell rings in their respective dining rooms, in the morning before breakfast, and in the evening before supper to hear read a portion of the Holy Scriptures and for prayers, they shall pay strict attention and behave in an orderly manner'*.

Article 12 states, *'All inmates shall be required to work either inside or outside the hospital, at such calling, or trade, and to take such care and do such work as they may be ordered to do, suitable to their age, sex, capacity, and state of health, under such penalties and such punishment as the Executive Committee may deem fit to inflict, in accordance with the disciplinary code adopted,'* but said inmates should have the right to appeal to the Directors.

One interesting regulation *'For warders and inmates of the lunatic asylum'* is contained in Article 3, *'The inmates shall go out in the grounds provided for their recreation for at least one hour during the morning, and for a longer period during the afternoon, according to the season of the year and the state of the weather, always under the supervision of the warders, and they should as much as possible be occupied or amused, it being well known that bodily occupation and mental amusement are objects of the first importance to those of unsound mind'*.

There is a very strict disciplinary code, the penalty for refusing to obey orders, using profane, or abusive language, refusing to work, drunkenness or smoking out of hours or in prohibited places included *"admonition for the first or second offence up to and including the seven days' cells. Should the term be for no more than 48 hours, the offender may be kept the whole time on bread and water, but if more than 48 hours, the offender can only be kept on bread and water on alternate days, the whole under the supervision of the Medical Officer".*

In 1918 after the First World War both the Town and Country Hospitals were taken over by the States of Guernsey. Their role was as public assistance institutions.

During the 1930's Lady Ruth Vene, the wife of the Lieutenant Governor took an intense interest in the unsatisfactory state of the Asylums at St Julians House (female) and the Country Hospital (male). The States Asylum Committee commissioned a report from Dr Saxby Good, described as *'a well known alienest of high repute'*. This report condemned the existence of these institutions in very emphatic language, equally emphatically advocating the building of an entire new mental hospital, and recommending the appointment of a specialist for a year at least, who would investigate the local provision as regards mental disease and deficiency and report to the Committee.

This report was accepted, and the States approved the construction of an up to date psychiatric hospital at Le Vauquiedor (now the Princess Elizabeth Hospital) and appointed Dr William McGlashan as the first 'States Mental Officer'.

However, because the new mental hospital had not yet been completed, Dr McGlashan agreed to undertake duties as schools medical officer as described in Chapter Seven.

In 1939 the Country Hospital was converted into an Emergency Hospital to deal with expected war casualties, as well as the full range of maternity, general, medical and surgical cases.

In 1940 the new purpose-built psychiatric hospital opened at the Vauquiedor and in the same year was taken over for use as a military hospital by the German Occupying Forces. Throughout the war, mental patients therefore continued to be cared for in the overcrowded accommodation of the Town and Country Hospitals.

In 1941 part of the Covent at Les Cotils was commandeered by the Health Services Officer for use as an overflow for the Town Hospital, whilst in 1945 following Liberation, the Board of Health took responsibility for all health matters including hospitals, but excluding St Peter Port Hospital, which remained the responsibility of the Public Assistance Authority Hospital Board until 1970.

A psychiatric service is established

The work carried out at the Emergency Hospital (Castel Hospital) during the war demonstrated the need for a General Hospital, and in December 1945 the States agreed to invite an advisory council to visit the island to advise on future health and hospital services. The report prepared by Dr G Bourne, Dr F Grundy, and Mr J A Beardsell was published in full as an appendix to the Billet d'Etat in April 1946. They recommended that a psychiatrist should be included in the rota of visiting specialists to the Island. *'It was deemed unlikely that there would be available to the island a psychiatrist of Consultant status. The Board of Health was therefore encouraged to persuade local practitioners to take steps to include amongst their number one or two medical men who had taken the Diploma in Psychological Medicine. These together with a visiting consultant would serve to cover the field'.*

Pre-war and indeed until the early 1950's there was very little drug treatment for psychiatric patients. Hyperactive and schizophrenic patients were sedated mainly with paraldehyde and barbiturates and given general medical care. Patients with dementia succumbed fairly rapidly to chest or other infections in those pre-antibiotic days.

The Psychiatric services were normally assigned to the Assistant Medical Officer of Health, who was in effect responsible for running all the services and for the patients' medical care. Dr McGlashan who had been deported to Biberach along with other British Nationals returned with them after the war. After he died, the post was held by Dr J Best who also died in office. Dr Doran, who had worked in the Colonial Medical Services, returned from doing general medicine in Fiji and was appointed and paid as a medical officer. Private patients were seen by a Consultant Psychiatrist from the UK, usually by Dr David Stafford-Clark who came over for a few days at a time. At the end of 1962, Dr Barbara Salisbury came to the island and was asked to provide locum for holidays. She was concerned to find a limited use of modern drugs and unmodified Electro-Convulsive Therapy being given. When Dr Doran was offered a post in Fiji early in 1964, Dr Salisbury agreed to a long-term locum.

It was at this stage that outpatient clinics began to be held at the Princess Elizabeth Hospital. Individual case notes were made up for each patient. Prior to this all patient notes were in a large leather-bound book in the Superintendent's office. Patients would have individual drug cards and prescriptions were to be made up at the Princess Elizabeth Hospital rather than the Castel staff issuing drugs from bulk supplies.

Dr Salisbury and the British Medical Association advised the Board of Health that it was essential to appoint Consultant Psychiatrists with responsibility for the psychiatric services of the island. In accordance with the final agreement Dr Tony Gumbrell was appointed. During this period, assessments were made of each individual patient, and case histories and notes made up. The majority of patients were de-certified, and became voluntary patients.

Mental health in the community

In 1965 the Corbinerie was acquired and the Guernsey Society for the Mentally Handicapped formed. In 1966 Dr Gumbrell left the island and Dr Salisbury continued as a locum as well as continuing her work with the Education Council.

In 1967 Dr Nigel Best was appointed and plans were drawn up for a new Occupational Therapy Department. A 'Mental Health Week' was started and regular open days initiated where the public were invited to inspect the hospital. A League of Friends was formed and a mini bus was purchased. In 1969, the 1939 *Mental Health Act* was amended. An adult training centre opened at The Mignot Training Centre and the old training centre at Floraville closed. In his annual report in 1969 Dr Best reported, *'due in no small measure to the provocative price of alcohol in the Bailiwick one sees many more cases of acute and chronic alcoholism in a year here than during the corresponding year period on the mainland'*.

1972 saw a decrease in the stigma of the Castel Hospital and the number of admissions and outpatients increased accordingly.

1974 also was the inauguration of the Guernsey Council of Alcoholism. Dr Best in his annual report noted the shortage of nursing staff, especially those who were qualified. *'However, we are losing many others, some married, with partners also possessing nursing qualifications who, because of the almost total lack of suitable housing arrangements on the island, take fright at the initial interview because no solid assurances on this problem can be given'*. This comment, of course, remains relevant to the present day.

The need for change

The 1980's proved a challenging time for the Castel Hospital and the Mental Health Services in general. In June 1982 an internal report indicated the need for many changes right across the board. In August 1982 there was a report on the visit to services provided for the mentally ill and mentally handicapped performed by the National Health Services Health Advisory Service. It concluded *' The Castel Hospital is not now suitable for modern psychiatric practice. In the short term, there should be an urgent programme of improvements in the long-stay wards at the Castel Hospital, furnishings, decorations, sanitary arrangements. Mentally handicapped patients should be moved out of wards as a priority to community based accommodation. A future site for an acute admission unit should be within the Princess Elizabeth Hospital site. A range of services for the mentally ill should be developed in the community'*.

A further report was commissioned by Overall & Aylott of the Dorset County Council Social Services Department in 1983 to review the training and recreational facilities for mentally handicapped people in the Bailiwick of Guernsey. This had a wide ranging impact on the development of services for the mentally handicapped or 'learning disabled' as they were to become.

In 1987 Lawrence Tennant of the British Psychological Society carried out a review of *'Psychology Services in Guernsey with particular reference to the Board of Health services to those with a mental handicap'*. This supported the previous report indicating the need for a second psychologist and recommended a growth to one psychologist per 15,000 population. A second psychologist for the learning disability service came in to post in March 1989.

In February 1992 a review of the Services for Mental Health on Guernsey was carried out by a team from the University of Southampton and the Wessex Regional Health Authority - the so called *'Thompson Review'*. This recommended the appointment of a Psychogeriatrician and the appointment of a full-time Child Psychiatrist. It also suggested replacing Oberlands House with small units and increasing the residential provision for learning disabilities service. Clinical audit was recommended as was a voluntary Day Care Centre for mild dementia in the community.

Plans for the future

In 1996 Robert Wiley retired after 15 years of senior management at the Castel Hospital and John Mackey was appointed as Director of Mental Health and Aged Care Services. During this year great difficulty was again experienced in recruiting and retaining sufficient trained and experienced mental health nurses.

In 1997 a strategic direction workshop was held and a long term vision of the future developments of the island's mental health services proposed. 1997 also saw the launch of the King's Fund Organisation Audit Accreditation Scheme. A computerised Patient Administration System and a clinical coding system also came into operation for the first time.

In his 1998 annual report John Mackey noted that *'The Castel Hospital is beginning to look very 'tired' and is no longer an acceptable environment in which to provide modern day mental health care. We are pleased to hear that redevelopment of the hospital is top priority of the President'*.

Recent plans approved by the States foresee that within the near future, the Castel Hospital will cease to function in its present form and will transfer to the site of the former Oberlands, adjacent to the Princess Elizabeth Hospital as was originally recommended in 1982. Most of the mental health services will then be centralised on one site adjacent to the Princess Elizabeth Hospital. High standards of patient care can then continue to develop well into the next millennium.

Main Sources

With thanks to Dr Barbara Salisbury and acknowledgements to the annual mental health reports.

Chapter Six

Looking after the learning disabled

Mrs Sylvia Hickman

In 1930, it was reported that 'such a competent body as the Mental Deficiency Committee estimates that the proportion of population mentally sub-normal (in Guernsey) *is no less than 10%'. This personal account captures what it was like to care for children with learning disabilities in the 1960s and ends optimistically with plans and hopes for the future.*

Reflections on Floraville 1962

From one of the upstairs windows of Vauvert Secondary School I could look down into the playground of the small school next door called 'Floraville'. The playground took up some of the space of the larger school. The playground wall wasn't very high and Vauvert pupils would call out over the wall. *'Do you want your ball back?'* A large young girl called Ernestine would be swinging high on a wooden swing which creaked back and forth.

It was early April and I had volunteered to spend a week working next door. I was about to leave school and I thought I could manage to look after mentally handicapped people. The first day as soon as I opened the front door I was confronted by a young girl who was screaming and trying to tear off her clothes.

Assembly was unusual, a Mrs Dorothy Burnard, a lady I had been introduced to previously, was playing *'All things bright and beautiful'* and a child was playing a cacophony of notes on the same piano but at the bass end. I tried to look normal and pretend that I was used to this sort of behaviour. An anthracite stove glowed dimly red and the room had that cokey smell and was a little stuffy.

The school comprised of two class-rooms and a small hall leading to the caretaker's flat above. To the left of the entrance was an oblong cloakroom with very small basins lining one wall, whilst toothbrushes and mugs and towels were arranged for the children's use. Satchels and coats hung on low pegs.

I was introduced to Isabel Kirby, the teacher I was to be assigned to. In those days I was called a trainee. My job started at 9 o'clock at the bus terminus. The bus drivers called it the *'milk run'*, and my duties began with picking up all the children, other than the few who came by taxi. It took an hour and it was with a sigh of relief I ushered everyone out of the bus and into the school. No one had been sick on the bus on that occasion.

Our aim in those days was to try and fit these children into a mode of behaviour which would be acceptable in everyday life. We also tried to simulate a workshop environment where they spent some time making flower boxes. I vividly remember when their enthusiasm knew no bounds being surrounded by boxes.

With the pocket money earned, shopping expeditions were arranged and an awareness of money and what it could buy was learned. There were all levels of attainment, from succeeding in doing up shoe-laces, and buttons on fly-fronts, managing zips and hoods, which all took endless patience.

The tray game was popular, an assortment of objects were put on a tray and the children took it in turns to remember how many things there were and what they were. The concept of time was hard for most to grasp. Dinner time at 12 o'clock was easy and going home time, but hours and days and weeks and months and years were difficult. It was truly amazing how they could decipher one another's speech, when you were having trouble understanding it *'Please miss Johnny wants to go to the toilet'* and many more problems were solved this way.

Some of the children had multiple disabilities, from epilepsy to behaviour problems. There were medical names for all of them, which I was to learn later. Self inflicted wounds was one such malady; frustration would build up in a child if he could not communicate his wishes, and he would lash out on himself by biting wrists and knuckles.

My interview for the job had gone disastrously wrong. From the minute I sat on the hard back cane seated chair, I had not only felt shy and nervous, but intimidated as well. Opposite me sat six people at a very long table covered with a wine red cloth, confronting me with their icy stares.

I remember the answers I gave were honest, so honest in fact it turned out that they gave me the job. One of the questions was, did I enjoy sport? Not very much, I had answered. Another asked would I be happy taking P.E? Oh yes, I replied enthusiastically, especially if it was rounders or netball which somehow I hadn't connected with sport at all.

Would I be prepared to deal with 'fits' and children being sick, and helping the older boys to the toilet? Yes, I answered unaware of any foreseeable problems. Some of the children were taller than I was and nearly as old. At fifteen I was mistaken for one of the pupils more than once.

A trip away to Weymouth

I had only been there a few months when it was decided to take the children away to Weymouth for a holiday. We stayed in one of the Victorian guest houses overlooking the Esplanade. Potted geraniums tumbled over window boxes. The proprietress was an elderly lady who loved cats; there were cats everywhere, asleep on chairs and on window ledges. It was no wonder there were cats hairs in the blancmange. The bedrooms were clean and comfy, but I ate enough paste sandwiches to last a lifetime. It was a long day beginning with supervising the cleaning of teeth and making of beds, helping some of the younger ones to dress themselves, helping at breakfast time and calming down anyone who was upset. A good method was to sing and soon there would be smiles instead of tears.

One poor individual, Sandy, never stopped asking when he was going home. I had to take his shoes away at night and say they were needed for the shoe cleaning person, and that he would have them in the morning. Unless this precaution was taken he went 'walkabout' at midnight, which meant a frantic search to find him. Usually it was only a matter of a hundred yards, but he got cunning and would slip out whilst you were busy.

The trip to the Cheddar Gorge was both fantastic and frightening. The children had to be counted in and out again. In between there were long dimly lit passageways a bit damp with dripping condensation. The coach ride out there had been relaxing and everyone seemed to have enjoyed it. The day out had been a great success. All too soon the adventure was over and it was time to return to Guernsey by the Weymouth ferry.

Other holidays were organised and one to Jersey is especially vivid. We sat on a beach braving the elements, and nearly being overcome by the powerful smell of drying seaweed. The guest house proprietors where we stayed could not have been more understanding, for one of the children had been incontinent in the night. If we had been told by the parents, we would have been able to put a rubber sheet down, just in case. However, we offered to pay for a new mattress.

Understanding the theory

I was asked to read books by Freud and Jung, so that I would clearly know the difference between mentally ill persons, and mentally handicapped persons. The books were heavy going for a fifteen year old. A visit to the Castel Hospital soon put me right on this important matter, as indoor barred doors were locked behind me. I soon realised during the visit the problems some of the people had. Some elderly ladies clutched dolls to their bosoms, and gently rocked them back and forth. Some sat with vacant stares and other went through the motions of sweeping floors and having imaginary conversations.

It was very carefully explained to me that Down's Syndrome children suffered from a defect of the chromosomes. Dr J L H Down, an English physician in 1896, was the first person to realise this cause of such a disability. The children affected could be damaged to a greater or lesser degree; sometimes they were bright as buttons, other times they had no speech or hardly any at all. Mongolism was used as a term to describe the characteristics and appearance of the child, after the Mongol race, whose appearance was felt to be similar.

Encephalitis was explained to me as an inflammation of the brain, usually caused by a viral infection. Babies who contracted this virus could be 'brain damaged'. Another child might suffer from cerebral palsy, which would make it difficult for them to communicate, and they would have no control over their muscles. Walking unaided would be very difficult for them.

It was very important to be able to deal with epilepsy and to see that the child came to no harm whilst having an attack. It was important to be able to place them in the 'recovery position', and to make sure their airway was kept clear, and so reassure the child when they came around that all was well.

The autistic child was difficult to deal with for they tended to disrupt the classroom with their unusual behaviour patterns of tapping things and very fidgety movements and high pitched shrieks. It was almost impossible to obtain eye contact with the child, as they seemed preoccupied and stared into space. Music seemed to be the only thing to which they sometimes responded. Shaking tambourines and banging drums seemed to help them when they were especially disturbed.

Dyslexia was known about - we would show someone their written name but in a mirror and they would recognise the shapes. Often letters would be written backwards but reading and writing were very difficult for most. We used flash cards on objects like chair, table and window, it was surprising how many words could be remembered this way, but stringing whole words together was something else. Occasionally, someone would be very good at numbers and if you told them your date of birth, somehow they could work out what day it was in an instant. Perhaps, in this sort of instance part of the brain was working superbly. They could add and subtract in a moment, but this was extremely rare to find a child such as this.

Further developments for the learning disabled

We moved from 'Floraville' to Maurepas School (now the Longfield Centre) and from there to Mont Varouf School. Sometimes the brighter children who were really borderline cases were moved to Valnord School. Deaf children were helped by being given a special classroom which was wired up especially so that they could take their lessons together.

Swimming lessons were very popular and once the fear of the water was overcome, it was difficult to get the children to come out of the water, so that the next class was able to use it. There was a playing field at Mont Varouf and pupils enjoyed football and outdoor activities, especially playing against other teams.

Cookery classes were also very popular and had been used to form basic skills in looking after yourself, as it was called. Electric kettles were filled, cups of tea made, ironing and all the everyday tasks we have to do and take for granted were shown to the young adults, who with supervision learned to be careful with boiling water and hot irons.

They laid tables for meals and were shown how to clean shoes and tidy up afterwards. They made baskets and simple wooden articles, and enjoyed fete days and open days when visitors and mums and dads would be looking at the children's work. Painting was always popular and model making and anything made with their hands. Some enjoyed growing things such as mustard and cress, and beansprouts would be watched closely for developments. This was developed if possible by encouraging trips to garden centres to see how things grew in greenhouses. With supervision an interest in greenhouse work could be obtained, and in this way it was hoped that sheltered workshops could be set up so that the young adult had a place to work safely when he or she left school.

The Reverend Mignot legacy was bequeathed to the States of Guernsey in 1935. When his wife died in 1962, La Corbinerie also became available to both the Board of Health and the Education Committee. It was decided that an adult rehabilitation and respite centre be set up. This was established on 1st September 1969. Now nearly thirty years later, much has changed as regard to the health and well being of the people with learning disabilities. The Mignot Centre and Interwork Services are there for the many who need individual attention.

There is a snooze room especially designed to put persons in a relaxed frame of mind. With the aid of soft music and moving coloured lights in tubes this can be achieved - a little like watching tropical fish at the dentist. The ambience of the place is one of informality. The rooms are light and airy and each individual chooses what he or she would like to do each day. There are well equipped kitchens and lunches can be prepared and eaten, whilst skills such as learning how to use coffee machines and a micro-wave oven can be obtained.

Outdoor workshops are available to simulate a 'nine to five' job, where the 'minimum allowance' is earned so as not to interfere with the benefits a person may be receiving already. This keeps things uncomplicated for the person with a learning disability. Sport and visits to swimming pools and places of local interest are encouraged. Literacy skills, money, time, local knowledge, and self-advocacy is made available enabling everyone who wishes to have a say in the running of the Mignot Centre a chance to air their views.

Whenever possible individuals are encouraged to live full lives independently in bed sits. Others may need long term care with a carer. Others are looked after at home by their parents, until the time comes for them to choose an independent life whenever possible.

Hope for the future

It is hoped that now new plans for improvements to the Mignot Centre have been approved by the States of Guernsey, it will enable the Centre to have a dining room where individuals don't have to put their coats and hats on in order to reach it in wet weather. It will make it so much easier if plans go through for a one level ground floor, where all bath aids and hoists will be made available for the physically disabled who need help. The small things which make the quality of life that little richer and gives the individual dignity, could perhaps include a cheerful hairdressing salon with pictures and flowers and magazines and coffee available, a place for a chat and a laugh, a place to be at ease in?

There are at present 212 people with a learning disability on the Services register. People of all ages and various degrees of learning disability can be helped, there are nine residential group homes providing long term care for 64 adults altogether.

Grow Limited was opened by Sir Charles Frossard on 14th July 1984. It provides a sheltered workplace for people with a learning disability. Some gardening work is also undertaken away from the workplace, such as mowing of lawns and contract work.

'Handicapped dancers succeed' made headlines in the local press, as did *"Trainees mastering their life skills course"*. Swimming gala success has come to many with a learning disability, who have worked hard and obtained fulfilment when a job or a challenge has been met with determination. Riding for the disabled has given confidence to those who need it most, and the reward has been the confidence in the children's faces after the lessons. Both helpers and participants have gained much from such experiences. A great deal of help is given in a voluntary way by many individuals, who give their time to the welfare of others, either by raising money for holidays, or helping organise leisure pursuits for the people with a learning disability. Many such go unacknowledged, but without their hard work, much progress in the care of people with a learning disability would not have been accomplished.

The Education Council have proposed plans to the States of Guernsey for a new school. It would incorporate such schools as Mont Varouf and the Longfield Centre, whose facilities are far from ideal. It would not only cater for children with a learning disability or children with a physical handicap, but would be able to help children with an eating disorder, or in some cases mental illness and some who felt stressed out with exam worries and family crises and concerns. It is hoped that physiotherapists and speech therapists will continue to visit the school and so cut down on lost schooling. All these children would benefit from larger purpose built premises.

Chapter Seven

Health Services for Children

Richard Hocart

Concern about the poor physical state of many Army recruits led to the establishment of the School Medical Services in Britain in the early years of this century. Other Nations, notably the United States and Germany quickly followed. Despite repeated calls for a School Medical Service in Guernsey, the first School Nurses were only appointed in 1927, and it was a further ten years before a part-time School's Medical Officer took up post. During the post war years, the Service has developed in complexity and range, to meet the changing health needs of different generations of students.

From 1900 to the Occupation Years

The twentieth century has seen a great improvement in the health of children in Guernsey, and like children elsewhere in the West, they have benefited enormously from advances in medical science and general improvements in the standard of living.

In 1901 there were 13,400 children under the age of 15 in Guernsey. Lack of means and, in some cases, parental ignorance denied many of them access to such medical services as were available to those children whose parents had means and education. Bodily defects, such as poor eyesight and hearing, went undetected and untreated, and undernourishment was not uncommon. It is interesting to note that, although Guernsey's population increased by 18,200 between 1901 and 1996, the number of children under the age of 15 in 1996 was 10,341 - fewer than in 1901. The change in the ratio of children to adults is due to a reduction in the average number of children born to each woman and greater longevity.

Compulsory education was introduced in Guernsey in 1901. All children between 5 and 13 were required to attend school. This brought children from well-run and hygienic homes into closer contact with those from less hygienic homes and increased the risk of transmission of disease and lice.

In the early years of the twentieth century outbreaks of dangerous contagious diseases were frequent. Diphtheria which was rare in Guernsey prior to 1895, claimed the lives of some children every year, and in many years epidemics of measles and scarlet fever took more young lives. Many more however caught these diseases and recovered, but they missed important schooling as a result, whilst contacts were also excluded from school until they had been declared free from infection. Occasionally so many children were absent that a school might be closed until the epidemic had passed. For example, measles led to the closure of several schools in 1920 and again in 1936. Tuberculosis was another cause of death in childhood, but most of the 40 or 50 deaths a year were amongst the adult population. However, smallpox had declined as a cause of death following compulsory vaccination for all infants introduced to Guernsey in 1896.

In 1906 Dr Henry Draper Bishop, the Medical Officer of Health, recommended that the States should appoint a School Medical Officer who would be responsible for inspecting all children in the elementary schools in order to detect physical defects and to advise parents how their children's health could be improved. His plea for action reflected a widely felt concern: *'At the present time, when so much is heard of the physical degeneration of our race, surely such a plan as this should be the foundation of our efforts to cope with this evil?* (MoH Annual Report for 1905).

Bishop's recommendation was ignored, but over the next three decades until his retirement in 1935 he undertook numerous school visits himself, usually to examine children whose condition was causing concern to the school staff. The Education Council, formed in 1916 from an amalgamation of three committees dealing with education, paid grants to enable children to have tonsils and adenoids removed and spectacles supplied.

A School Health Service starts

In 1926 Bishop again recommended that a School Medical Officer be appointed, and also advised that two school nurses and a school dentist were needed. Guernsey now lagged behind England, where all local education authorities had been required since 1921 to provide a school medical service. This time, his advice was followed - at least in part. In 1927 the Education council appointed two part-time nurses to carry out inspections and to deal with minor ailments.

One of these nurses resigned in the following year and the other, Mrs Pattison, was appointed to a full-time post. The Council appointed a Medical Committee of four members to supervise her work. Mrs Pattison served the Council until her retirement in 1955. A second school nurse was appointed in 1937.

The appointment of the first School Medical Officer was an indirect consequence of a States decision to improve the treatment of mental illness. In 1933, Dr William McGlashan was appointed on a one year contract, later made permanent, as the States Mental Officer. The duties attached to this post were insufficient to occupy him full time, especially as proposals to build a mental hospital were not immediately put into effect, and in 1935 the States agreed that McGlashan would also be a part-time School Medical Officer under the direction of the Education Council. The *Loi Relative à la l'Instruction Primaire* of 1935 made it a responsibility of the Council to organise the medical inspection, and treatment of elementary school children.

McGlashan's annual reports record the results of his medical inspections. For example, in 1936 he saw 121 children who needed to be referred for treatment to their family doctor and 110 who needed to be seen by the two Ophthalmic Specialists then working in the island. Financial assistance was obtained from various sources when families could not afford treatment. Twenty-eight children, some requiring orthopaedic treatment in England, were helped by the Children's Aid Society. Twenty-nine families were advised to seek help from the Poor Law Board. Other families were assisted by the Education Council.

The 1935 report explained that the Council was only recommended to give aid *'to those cases who from inquiry appeared to be incapable financially of procuring adequate medical attention and who for obvious reasons hesitated to ask for Poor Law Relief'*. These were probably families who were on the borderline for Poor Law assistance and were just managing to maintain their independence.

McGlashan and the School Nurses operated a Minor Ailments Clinic and dispensed medicine to children with such ailments. Parents were encouraged to attend when their children were inspected and they were advised about hygiene and general child care. McGlashan urged the Council to provide hot water in school lavatories; his successors were still waging this battle twenty years later. McGlashan also reported that boys under 16 had easy access to cigarettes and urged the authorities to enforce the law which made it an offence to sell tobacco products to children under 16.

The poor physical condition of quite a large number of schoolchildren caused the Education Council concern. With States approval, the Council introduced a *'Milk in Schools'* scheme in 1935. Every elementary school child was entitled to a third of a pint of milk each day. Those who could afford to pay were charged 1/2d a day, while those who could not pay received their milk free of charge. The headteacher at the Vale School weighed his boy pupils periodically and found that those who took milk gained more weight than those who did not. The Council provided each school with a weighing machine so that the progress of all pupils could be monitored.

In 1938 there was a widespread outbreak of diphtheria. The Board of Health ran a voluntary immunisation scheme, and just over 50% of the children were immunised. Many parents positively refused to have their children immunised. McGlashan and Dr Rowan Revell, the Medical Officer of Health, advocated compulsory immunisation. The States agreed that compulsion was required and passed the necessary legislation in 1938, but implementation was delayed by the war and the law was not brought into force until 1949.

The Occupation Years

Following the invasion of France in May 1940, and the rapid advance of the German army, 5,200 school children were evacuated to England, some with their parents but the majority without. 1,050 school children remained in Guernsey and from 30th June found themselves under German rule. Many children under school age also remained in Guernsey with their families, so the school population gradually increased during the Occupation. By the time of the Liberation there were 1,550 pupils in the schools. Most of the school buildings were requisitioned by the Germans, and the Council was obliged to lease halls and private houses for schools.

McGlashan remained in Guernsey in 1940, but the two school nurses, Mrs Pattison and Miss Eardley, left for England. McGlashan maintained a programme of school medical inspections and the local District Nursing Association took on the responsibility of inspecting children for lice and minor ailments.

In September 1942 McGlashan was among a large number of island residents deported to internment camps in southern Germany. Regular medical inspection of school children was suspended.

Scarcity of food affected the health and educational performance of school children during the Occupation years. The causes were, of course, beyond the control of the Education Council and the States, but the Council did what it could to ensure that the children received adequate nourishment. The *'Milk-in-Schools'* Scheme continued to operate, and by 1943 nearly every child was taking advantage of it. A number of communal kitchens were also opened around the island, and wherever possible, pupils received a hot mid-day meal subsidised by the Council.

By late 1943 the physical condition of the children was deteriorating. Children were weighed regularly in school, and the Education Council's annual report, written in February 1944, records that between December 1943 and January 1944 25% of the children lost weight, and that between January and February 33% lost weight. The situation deteriorated further towards the end of 1944 when the Channel Islands were cut off and besieged. Starvation was prevented by the arrival of Red Cross food parcels, brought by the *'Vega'*, which first came on 27th December and then returned at monthly intervals.

After the Liberation

Guernsey was liberated on 9th May 1945. During the next four months the children who had been evacuated without their parents returned home. Family relationships had to be rebuilt, and habits and values acquired in foster homes had to be accommodated or modified. Many of the families who had chosen to leave together in 1940 also returned. By September 1946 there were 5,877 children attending school in Guernsey.

Dr McGlashan, who had worked as a Medical Officer in an internment camp for Channel Islanders at Biberach, returned in 1945, as did the two school nurses.

Over the next twenty years the health services provided by the Education Council and the Board of Health for island children were gradually extended. The pace at which the services were developed is shown by a brief summary of what was achieved.

In 1950 the Board appointed two health visitors, one of whose duties was to monitor the health and development of pre-school children. In the same year the Board established an orthoptic service. Tuberculin testing for tuberculosis was introduced in 1953 and an immunisation programme for tuberculosis was started by the Board in 1955 using the BCG vaccine. (The vaccine's full name is Bacillus Calmette-Guerin. Two French scientists, Calmette and Guerin discovered the organism which produces a resistance to tuberculosis.) The School Dental Service was inaugurated in 1955 and in the following year the Council provided physiotherapy for asthmatics and speech therapy for the first time. The Board launched a voluntary programme of inoculation against poliomyelitis in 1957. The Council introduced a psychiatric service, the Child Guidance Clinic in 1963.

(The School Medical Service was essentially a single child health service and was presented as such in the School Medical Officer's annual reports, but it was also the practice to refer to the each part as a 'service', for example: the Speech Therapy Service. The whole Service was often referred to as the School Medical Services reflecting its character as a group of specialist services provided by two committees.)

By 1950 it was clear to the Board and the Council that McGlashan's role as Medical Superintendent, Mental Health Services, as it was styled, was becoming a full-time job, and it was decided that a new post of Assistant Medical Officer of Health should be created. The postholder would undertake the work of the School Medical Officer, and would also assist the MoH in his other public health work.

McGlashan died in office at the end of 1950, and Dr Doris Fox acted as temporary School Medical Officer, pending the appointment of an Assistant MoH/SMO. No suitable candidates applied for the post in 1951, and it was not until the summer of 1952 that Dr J P O'Riordan was appointed. He decided to leave in October 1952.

Before a successor was appointed the Board of Health and the Education Council agreed that the School Medical Officer should be responsible to the Medical Officer of Health and through him to the Council, thereby establishing that the Medical Officer of Health had overall professional responsibility for the School Medical Services.

Dr O'Riordan's successor, Dr Philip Murphy served from 1953 to 1954, and he was followed in turn by Dr F R N Lynch (1954-57, who then became MoH), Dr Charles McKeagney (1957-59) and Dr Margaret Liddell (1960).

'Eyes and teeth'

In 1955 the Education Council handed over responsibility for the appointment and supervision of the school nurses to the Board of Health. The Board recruited nurses who were qualified to work as health visitors, and by 1961 the Board had established a unified system of health visitors/school nurses. Later the roles were separated again.

Financial help towards the cost of eye examinations by a specialist and the supply of spectacles had been part of the pre-war School Medical Services. In 1946 Dr Martin opened an ophthalmic practice in Guernsey, but the Council found that it was cheaper to engage an eye specialist from Jersey to conduct a regular eye clinic for school children in Guernsey. In 1947 Dr Frank Neubert came to Guernsey and was engaged by the Council to examine children under the Service, to prescribe spectacles and to perform squint operations. Dr Neubert worked as the local ophthalmic surgeon for 27 years, before retiring in 1974. Drs Robin and Barbara Bonner-Morgan took over the practice, followed by Dr Richard Reynolds.

In January 1948 Dr Neubert met the Education Council and explained that if the ophthalmic service was to be effective it was essential to have an orthopist, who would provide the necessary therapy to correct mild squints and to complete the development of binocular vision after operations. The Board of Health, agreed that, as the health of pre-school children was the Board's responsibility and as many of the children requiring orthoptic treatment would be pre-school children, the orthoptist should be a member of the Board's staff.

The States approved the creation of the post, and in 1950 the Board appointed Mrs Mary Edwards, who worked as the States orthoptist until her retirement in 1983. As the Board was short of accommodation, the Orthoptic Clinic was established in the Education Office at La Porte. In 1956, when access to the whole School Medical Service was extended to pre-school children, the orthoptist was transferred to the staff of the Education Council.

In 1962 the Medical Officer of Health, Dr Thomas, looking back on the ophthalmic work carried out in Guernsey, wrote: *'During the past few years it has emerged that Squint and Visual Defects are a major problem in this Island. In fact one child in seven suffers from some eye defect or other. This is probably largely due to hereditary influences, but the position has been aggravated by the fact that such defects often manifest themselves before school age and even if they develop later are not always picked up by routine examination'*. (Education Council Annual Report 1962). Eight years later his successor, Dr White recorded progress in his annual report: *'Mrs Edwards mentions that hardly ever does she see a school entrant with a visible squint thanks to the work of the health visitors of this Island'*. (Education Council Annual Report 1970).

The establishment of a School Dental Service was long delayed by setbacks. The original decision to establish a service was taken by the Education Council in 1938, but the plan was abandoned when war broke out. In 1946 the Council invited Dr A T Wynne, a Dental Officer at the Ministry of Education, to advise on the establishment of a dental service. He recommended that the Council needed two dentists to cover all the school children and might need a third in due course. The Council decided to start with one, but delayed seeking States approval owing to lack of accommodation and a reported shortage of dentists in the United Kingdom. Dr Wynne found that the children's dental health was generally good, particularly so in the case of those who had been in Guernsey during the Occupation.

The Council submitted its proposal to employ a dentist to the States in 1953. The proposal was accepted, and the States agreed that the service should be available to all the pupils in the States schools, including the Intermediate Schools. A dentist was appointed but was unable to take up his post owing to ill-health. While the post was being re-advertised, Mr F M Kay, a dentist in private practice, carried out a survey among local children and found that the incidence of decay was much higher than in England.

Eventually in 1955 Mr G J Ellis took up the post of School Dentist, and early in 1956 the School Dental Clinic opened at Lukis House. Ellis left for personal reasons after four months in post, and was succeeded by Miss Kathleen Beamish, who served until 1961. It proved impossible for one dentist to provide a comprehensive service, and in 1960 a second dentist, Mr R C R Eve was appointed. Both dentists left in 1961. Dr Thomas paid tribute in his annual report to Miss Beamish's 'excellent work' in organising and delivering dental treatment. She was succeeded by Mr Donal Hearns, and Mr Ronald Gregory was appointed as Assistant School Dental Officer. Under Mr Hearns the service began to offer orthodontic treatment (to straighten poorly aligned teeth). In 1969 the Clinic moved to La Couperderie, where the Education Office was located following its move from La Porte, and a third dentist was appointed.

'School milk'

The pre-war *'Milk-in-Schools'* scheme, which the Council had managed to keep going during the Occupation, was suspended at the end of the war. Before the war school milk had been delivered in bottles which were returned and washed, but after the war the Dairy had no facilities for washing bottles. (Householders provided their own jugs to receive milk delivered from door to door). After the war the Board of Health ran a scheme for subsidising the cost of milk supplied to households on low incomes. In 1951 the States decided that the Board should cease to operate the scheme and directed the Essential Commodities Committee to organise a scheme for the provision of free milk at home to children and expectant mothers in low income households.

Headteachers were concerned at the absence of a supply of milk in school and in 1953 they urged the Council to re-introduce the pre-war scheme. The Council decided against this measure, partly because a convenient system of packaging milk was not available, but also because no cases of malnutrition had been brought to its attention. Dr Murphy, the newly appointed Assistant School Medical Officer, investigated the condition of the school children and informed the Council in his annual report for 1953 that *'4.3% [of the children examined] fall into the category of "poor general condition" (comparable figure for England and Wales in 1951 was 2.9%). This figure is too high; it can be reduced to some extent, in my opinion, by the immediate re-introduction of bottled milk in schools. This will ensure that the children in most need of it will get it. I feel that at the present one has no guarantee that the child recommended for cheap milk is receiving it and that it is not pooled with the family supply'*.

On receiving this report, the Bailiff, Sir Ambrose Sherwill, asked the Council if something could be done for these children? As a result of the Bailiff's intervention the Council and the Red Cross devised a scheme for the supply of milk, eggs, cod liver oil and malt to undernourished children identified by the Assistant School Medical Officer. The Council, with States approval, provided the necessary funds.

In 1959 the States agreed that children in poor physical condition could, on the recommendation of the Assistant School Medical officer, receive a free half pint of milk a day in school. This scheme was intended to help those who were not in so poor a state as those classed as undernourished. Owing to the illness and departure of Dr McKeagney, the milk scheme was not launched until 1961.

Further changes

In the 1950's developments in the School Medical Service were delayed by frequent staff changes. In 1960 Dr A Thomas became Medical Officer of Health and Schools Medical Officer. He handed over in 1969 to Dr Geoffrey White, who had served as his deputy for some years. Dr White was head of the Service for 14 years. He was assisted from 1965 by Dr Elizabeth Witherick, who assumed responsibility for the day to day running of the Service in 1969, when she became Deputy School Medical Officer. She retired in 1984. Under the long and dedicated leadership of these doctors the Service achieved a new level of effectiveness.

Dr Thomas reorganised the school nurses and health visitors in 1962, combining the two services, but separate school nurses were re-introduced by Dr White. Inspections for head-lice continued to be part of the school nurses' duties. Until the 1960's the head of the infected child was treated with a sticky emulsion of Benzyl benzoate, which had to be kept on for 24 hours and had an unpleasant smell. A shampoo was introduced in 1964. This proved to be much more acceptable, and a decrease in infections was soon noticed.

Thomas realised the importance of health education, and advised the Education Council that every school should have a health education syllabus. In 1963, when the link between smoking and lung cancer had finally been confirmed, the Council agreed to fund an anti-smoking campaign in the schools, and a health education exhibition was held at the Grammar Schools. Thomas and Hearns advocated fluoridation of the water supply to combat dental decay, but as Thomas reported in 1963, the idea met *'stolid opposition'* and was temporarily abandoned.

A part-time speech therapy service was begun in 1956. The first speech therapist was Miss E Le M Foard, who operated in rented rooms in the Grange Road. Her case-load increased from 49 children in 1957 to 83 in 1961. When she left in 1963 the post was made full-time and the Clinic moved to Granville House in Mount Durand. Miss Foard's successor was Miss J F Alexander (1963-64), followed by Miss Jenny Richmond (1965-1996).

Successive School Medical Officers from McGlashan onwards advised the Education Council to provide special education for children with disabilities. The first special school opened by the Council was Floraville, established in 1948 for about 12 children with severe mental handicaps. Five years later the school moved to Valnord, where a larger number of children (with various disabilities) could be accommodated. The creation of Valnord and the speech therapy service ended the era when the parish school had to teach disabled children without any external or specialised support.

The Child Guidance Clinic

In 1963 the Council decided to employ a psychiatrist on a part-time basis. Dr Barbara Salisbury agreed to establish a Child Guidance Clinic. In the first few years of its existence 35 to 50 new cases a year were referred to Dr Salisbury. A social worker was appointed to undertake the associated social work, which involved many home visits. Initially the Clinic was held at Lukis House, but, owing to lack of a suitable room and the reluctance of some parents to bring their children to a building used by various services, the Clinic moved to Dr Salisbury's home, where it remained until 1991, when alternative accommodation was found, first at a doctors' surgery and then at the Princess Elizabeth Hospital.

As some of the children referred to the Child Guidance Clinic were living at the Children's' Home or came from families being monitored by the Children Board or the National Society for the Prevention of Cruelty to Children (NSPCC), it was necessary to develop close links with the Board. Co-ordination was improved through a 'Problem Families Investigation Committee' established in 1967 by the Education Council.

The needs of children with impaired hearing were brought to the Council's attention by Miss Jessie de Garis, the first headteacher of Valnord School, and later the first educational psychologist employed by the Council. There was no system of testing to detect impaired hearing among infants, and virtually no special tuition for those children who were known to have a hearing problem. The Council appointed a teacher of the deaf, Mr Roger Goldsmith, in 1970 to establish a testing programme, to give special tuition and to provide advice about hearing aids. In 1971 Mrs Joan Goodwin was appointed to conduct audiometric tests.

Other innovations in this period were the introduction of immunisation against German Measles (rubella) in 1972 and measles in 1981, and remedial physiotherapy for handicapped pupils.

The School Medical Services were open from 1956 to all pre-school children and all school-children except feepayers at Ladies' College and Elizabeth College and the private schools. Most of the services provided directly by the Council were free of charge. (Charges were made for speech therapy and physiotherapy until 1970.) The costs of treatment provided by private practitioners (ENT and ophthalmic treatment, spectacles and hearing aids) were recovered from parents according to a sliding scale related to income, with the poorest families paying nothing.

Despite the fact that some of the staff within the Services were accountable to the Education Council for their School Medical work and to the Board of Health for other duties, the Services functioned smoothly in the 1960's and 1970's. By the 1980's there was a perceived need for more strategic planning of health services and of state assistance for families paying medical bills. In 1985, at the invitation of the Board, a team of medical experts, led by Sir Douglas Black, prepared a report on health care in Guernsey. The Black Committee was, no doubt, influenced by the fact that education authorities in England had ceased to be responsible for the medical inspection and treatment of school children. The Committee described the Education Council's involvement in the provision of health care as *'anomalous'* and recommended that this responsibility should be transferred to the Board of Health.

The Board of Health takes over

Discussions took place between the Council and the Board about a transfer of responsibility. A number of issues had to be resolved, including future accommodation for the different clinics and the way in which medical and education staff would work together when the Board assumed responsibility. Eventually agreement was reached and in February 1988 the States agreed the Board should become responsible for the Services. A change in the law transferred the Council's statutory responsibility to organise the medical inspection and provision of treatment of pupils to the Board, and on 1st January 1989, the Board of Health assumed responsibility for the Services.

When Dr Witherick retired in 1984, Dr Desmond Creery agreed to come out of retirement to act as Senior Clinical Medical Officer. He was succeeded by Dr Neil Boyle, who was appointed as Guernsey's first Consultant Community Paediatrician.

With the move to 'Child Health Services', feepaying pupils were given access to the Services. The Social Security Authority assumed administrative responsibility for aiding families who could not afford the fees for their children's medical treatment.

The Orthoptic Clinic, the Speech Therapy Clinic and the Dental Clinic were moved to the Princess Elizabeth Hospital. Today the Speech and Language Clinic has a staff of six therapists who work with children and adults of all ages. The Dental Clinic employs three dentists, a dental therapist and a dental hygienist. Psychiatric services for children and adolescents are now based at Bell House in the Grand Bouet.

Plans for the future

In 1999, following the retirement some two years before of Dr Boyle, the Medical Specialist Group agreed to provide a community paediatric service for the Board of Health. Now the Group's three paediatricians will provide the medical inspection and referral service begun by the Education Council in 1935. The Group also provides the audiology screening services as part of the their paediatric service. The monitoring and developmental check-ups of pre-school children and school children continue to be provided by the Board health visitors and school nurses.

At the end of the twentieth century children in Guernsey face far less risk of catching life-threatening infectious diseases than did their great grand-parents 100 years ago. Children are taller and better nourished, and physical defects are now rare. Physical maturity also comes much earlier than it did in 1900, whilst defects of sight can often be overcome by therapy and surgery, and much can be done to assist children with impaired hearing.

But today's children also face health risks. Death from meningitis can still occur with little warning, but fortunately this is uncommon. HIV and AIDS are new risks for young adults. The prevalence of childhood asthma is steadily increasing, and drug use and dependency has also increased. Family break-down also imposes new stresses, especially in an island community.

Main Sources:

Much of the material in this chapter can be found in the published annual reports of the Education Council and the School Medical Officers. I must thank the Council for access to its records, Dr Barbara Salisbury for information about the Child Guidance Clinic and present members of the Child Health Services for patiently answering my requests for information.

Chapter Eight

The Community Nursing Service

Anne Jones

For the great part of this century, most births and deaths and much medical care took place outside hospital, in people's homes and in other community settings. Essential to the delivery of this care were the nurses of the three Guernsey District Nursing Associations. The contribution of community nurses, and the increasing specialisation of their roles forms the theme of this chapter.

A rich history ....

At its centenary the Board of Health can be proud of its excellent community nursing service. This includes District Nurses, School Nurses, Health Visitors and Specialist Nurses, with knowledge and skills to provide nursing care for those who may need it because of terminal illness, problems with continence management, or other special needs in the community.

Today's community nurses continue to provide a service to patients outside the hospital setting. This can be in their own homes, in clinics, in schools, or in other settings which are accessible to them. Irrespective of the place of delivery, the focus of community nursing care is always on the individual patient or client, their carers and family. The aim of care is always to meet the needs of those patients or clients who are referred to the service, and thus come into contact with the nurses concerned.

Community nursing today has been built on a solid foundation - that sterling work which was undertaken by nurses in the local communities on the island during the early part of the century, through the war years and beyond. Indeed the history is rich.

This chapter traces some of this early history. It highlights milestones, and illustrates some of the most important developments. The issues outlined in the chapter are key components in the contribution of the community nursing service to the steadily improving health of the island's people. These include social change and attitudes to care, the registration of nurses, the development of district nursing, the early organisation of Guernsey's community nursing service, the responsibilities of the District Nursing Associations and more recent developments in community nursing to the millennium and beyond.

Social change and attitudes to care

Nursing has developed in response to changing social needs. As the structure of society has altered, so new demands for health care have arisen. New habits and customs influence disease patterns whilst changes in the size and composition of the population create new problems.

These problems are continuing and tend to accelerate as knowledge accumulates, but they are also to an extent unpredictable. During some periods development seems so slow that variation is almost imperceptible. At other times circumstances combine to produce change so quickly that the whole social basis alters in one generation. The corollary of this is that with rapid changes come new ideas about 'rights' and responsibilities, and indeed the whole social purpose. Although opinions differ as to what is fundamental to social change, there is no doubt that the pattern of society changes and, as it does so it produces new health needs in the community. Social change and subsequent changing attitudes to care therefore provide a backcloth to any health care service development, of which community nursing is no exception.

The registration of nurses

Formal training for nurses in hospitals has been available in Britain since the late 1880's. At that time there was conflict within nursing regarding the need for registration. In 1889, a mass meeting called for an official register of nurses who had completed an approved programme of training, but nothing was to come of this for some years.

In 1904 the National Council of Nurses of the United Kingdom was formed, but despite much lobbying and campaigning, formal registration only occurred at the end of 1919 when the *'Nurses Bill'* was approved by Parliament. As a result, a General Nursing Council for England and Wales was established, with the responsibility of setting up a Register of Nurses.

The register was to hold the names of those nurses who had completed a recognised programme of training and who satisfied the conditions of admission to one of the parts of the register - designated as general nursing, mental health nursing, sick children's nursing, or 'other', for example infectious diseases and fever nursing. There was also a separate part of the register for male nurses.

The issue of the registration of nurses is mentioned for two reasons, firstly until the late 1960's all qualified nurses working in Guernsey had had to leave the island to train for their qualification which was essential to gain their registration. Secondly, current registration with an individual's professional organisation is an explicit standard of quality, and today is actually the pre-requisite for employment in a professional capacity on the island.

District Nursing

The idea of the sick being cared for in institutions is, except in cases of extreme indigence, a comparatively modern one. From the diaconate of St Paul to St Vincent's Sisters of Mercy, emphasis has always been placed on the importance of providing care in the home. The move to care in hospitals came only when medical technology became too sophisticated for domestic application.

Although there have always been nurses visiting patients in their own homes, the modern concept actually dates from an experiment set up by Mr William Rathbone and Florence Nightingale in Liverpool in 1861, and the founding of the Queen Victoria Jubilee Institute in 1887. The Queen's Institute was a voluntary organisation run by local District Nursing Associations which collected subscriptions and donations. As time went by, the Queen's Institute was increasingly used by local authorities in the UK to provide a home nursing service. Different authorities had different practices, and some used other organisations, but it is a good example of statutory authorities taking over a service pioneered by a voluntary organisation.

This background to the history of district nursing is significant because the Guernsey District Nursing Associations were closely linked to the Queen's Institute for the validation of their local standards of practice.

The District Nursing Associations

Community nurses in Guernsey were based in the parishes and were part of an organisation known as the District Nurses Association (DNA). There were three District Nurses Associations in St Peter Port, St Sampson and the Vale, and 'the Country'.

The title 'nurse' was used collectively to describe both qualified State Registered Nurses, and the unqualified junior staff at the hospital. In the community however, nurses had to rely on the voluntary assistance and help of informal carers, who were usually family members and relatives of their patients.

Community nurses were employed by the respective District Nursing Associations, which was funded from parish funds, membership fees, and fees paid by patients. They also relied on other sources of income which came from donation, fund raising events, and interest on the Association's investments. Fees for maternity services were an additional source of income.

Nurses as members of the Association also paid an annual subscription.

Qualification for Community Nurses

The community nurses in the District Nurses Associations were qualified State Registered Nurses and were able to use the title SRN. Some were also State Certified Midwives and could then use the additional title 'SCM'.

At that time, and indeed for some considerable time later, midwifery training was of one year duration. Full qualification was awarded on completion of two discrete six month midwifery training programmes, both assessed at the end by a written and a practical examination. These were available at maternity hospitals, and in the maternity units of some of the larger British hospitals.

These midwifery programmes led to what were known as the Central Midwives Board (CMB) Part One, and Part Two qualifications. It was possible to complete the Part One programme only and to receive recognition by certification for this. Many nurses chose this option and subsequently they were then able to use the title SRN. CMB. (Part 1).

This information is shared here because the qualifications held by community nurses determined their participation in maternity care. Perhaps it was not seen as a quality indicator then, but it does demonstrate how nurses strove to maintain the safest standards for the community they served.

It must be remembered that as described in Chapter One, many women practising as midwives in Guernsey at this time had little training and no formal qualifications whatsoever. This was to lead to unacceptable levels of maternal mortality, and the eventual passage of the *'Ordonnance ayant rapport aux Sages Femmes'*, in 1936, which allowed the 'midwife' to summon medical assistance at no direct cost a poor women in labour. This was to have an important impact on reducing maternal mortality, but it was to be some years yet before all 'midwives' were required to be seek official registration.

Community nurses' roles and responsibilities

The community nurses provided care to all groups in the community including children, older people and maternity care. Each District Nursing Association nurses worked within their geographical areas but a 'holiday nurse' also worked across the boundaries providing relief cover as workload required.

The community nurses with full midwifery qualifications could provide maternity care for women and attend them in childbirth as autonomous practitioners. Those nurses with just the CMB Part One qualification could attend women and deliver the baby under the supervision of a fully qualified midwife.

The community nurses were able to go into the maternity hospital to deliver the women and take part in some of the hospital care. There was actually a scheme set up which allowed a hospital delivery and an early discharge home. This scheme was an innovative one for its time, and a predecessor of the early discharge plans which are implemented as part of maternity care offered today.

As the community nursing service developed so its workload increased. Some members of the District Nursing Associations began to realise that to continue to work as independent Associations was not as cost effective as working as a centralised resource could be. The aim of the service was to be able to meet the future health needs of the Guernsey population. It was therefore suggested that the three amalgamate, and a meeting was arranged to discuss this.

The Central Council of Guernsey District Nursing Associations

On April 15th 1935 an inaugural meeting of the Central Council of Guernsey District Nursing Associations was held at the Deanery. It was agreed that the Central Council would meet bi-annually, with additional meetings called as necessary. It was also agreed was that an Annual General Meeting would be held to elect an Honorary Chair, Secretary and Treasurer.

The Objects of the Central Council were:

   a. *'To promote co-operation in the island District Nursing Services and in liaison with the Queen's Institute of District Nursing*

   b. *To meet regularly to discuss all matters of interest relating to the services and take action as agreed;*

   c. *To consult with appropriate authority as required to ensure that home nursing and midwifery and other public services are related to each other'.*

The membership of the Central Council was made up of three nurses from each Association who were working officers, the Chair and Honorary Secretary and additional members with no voting powers. The Chair had the casting vote, and the Council had the power to co-opt up to three additional members to act in an advisory capacity, but without the power to vote. A visitor from the Queen's Institute of District Nursing could attend meetings, but with no voting power.

The annual membership subscription was agreed at £2 per member.

Voluntary help played a significant part in the community nurses work and they openly acknowledged this and urged that it continue. The input of volunteers was especially invaluable in child welfare clinics where community nurses would provide physical checks and advice on development and commonailments. A Board of Health publication *'To Mothers and Fathers - How to keep Yourselves and Your Children Well and Strong'* was available at sixpence (post free).

Collectively the Central Council generated income to help fund the community nursing service. There are records of £159 being raised from a 'Vanishing Teas Scheme' and £102 from a 'Bring and Buy Sale'. This money was shared equally between the three District Nursing Associations.

One of the objects of the Central Council was to ensure *'other public services are related to each other'*. This did have an impact when the Education Council contacted the Central Council to discuss the provision of free milk to children of pre-school age. It is clear that the community nursing service played a significant role in supporting the population in both illness and health in active and preventative measures. In so doing the nurses worked across the boundaries of the roles of midwives, nurses and health visitors.

There were no records of the Central Council meetings during the war years, but in 1948 the Central Council estimated the cost of a single nurse's visit to be three shillings and nine pence. In order to address the increasing cost of care and raise some extra funding, it was agreed to increase the nurses' subscription fee to the Association.

In 1949 the Central Council looked at the training of community nurses and proposed that one SRN be trained as a District Nurse and one as a Health Visitor. This was to be funded by the Central Council. Also this year the annual visit of the Queen's Institute Inspector took place.

During the early post war period there was an increase in the prevalence of tuberculosis amongst the island population. This had a serious impact on the work of community nurses, as the treatment required the administration of drugs by injection, with rest on the part of the patient. In order to manage this new demand, in 1959 the Board of Health awarded the Central Council a grant so that they could continue with their treatment and care of patients with tuberculosis.

The Board also assisted the community nursing service with money for the pads required by incontinent patients. It is clear that although community nursing was independent of the Board of Health in its formative years, the Board did in fact work closely with the service.

The service was developing and growing and the community nurses and their respective associations were well aware of this. Social changes coupled with escalating operating costs led to consideration of further Board of Health involvement.

Involvement of the Board of Health

Talks with the Board of Health about a possible handover had began in 1973. After careful discussion the Central Council reached the consensus that it would be in the interests of the District Nursing Service and the island if the Board of Health assumed responsibility. It was therefore proposed:

'That the States of Guernsey Board of Health be requested to take over the operation of the three District Nursing Associations'.

In 1975 the Central Council commissioned the building of a clinic at Lukis House in St Peter Port as a base for community nursing, whilst the details of terms and conditions for transfer were agreed.

The last meeting of the Central Council took place on 7th November 1977. The responsibility for the provision of the community nursing service from then on lay with the Board of Health.

The three District Nursing Associations donated their building at Lukis House as the focal point of the Board's District Nursing activities. A plaque to commemorate this is still on display there.

The role of Health Visitors in Community Nurses

The first health visitors employed by the Board of Health were able to practice in their own right rather than as generic community nurses. This meant that their practice was dedicated to the roles of health education, health promotion and health maintenance. All health visitors were qualified nurses with an additional community nursing specialist qualification in health visiting/public health nursing.

A health visitor today may first come into contact with a family at antenatal parentcraft classes and remain their contact after the birth of the baby and during the pre-school years. This close contact with individual families provides a continuity of care to a population which is not actually ill, and who can then make better informed choices about their own lifestyle and that of their dependants.

Health visitors also work with specific groups in the community like children suffering from problems such as eczema or asthma, but as well as their contact with individuals and their families, health visitors also work on wider community health issues. They can measure the positive benefits of their work in child accident prevention, breast feeding rates and immunisation and vaccination uptake.

School nursing

School nurses are also part of the community nursing service and work specifically with school age children in their respective school communities. The school nurse undertakes health interviews in school and is in a prime position to lead on health education initiatives on the school premises.

School nursing is a specialist branch in community nursing. As children are staying at school longer, school nurses have the opportunity to target the school population on health related issues such as exercise, healthy diet, sexual health, personal assertiveness and confidence building.

In keeping with the Central Council's previous objective, school nurses are well placed to ensure that their service is *'related to other public services in order to meet the needs of the area'*. School nurses work in close liaison with teachers and with the Education Council. They are in an excellent position to develop collaborative partnerships with colleagues to achieve the most effective outcomes in the health of school children and young people.

Community nursing in the home/district nursing

District nurses have faced a maelstrom of change with early discharge from hospital, increased longevity and the use of sophisticated equipment in the home. Added to this the use of powerful drugs has called for new skills and further training. The role of the district nurse continues to expand and develop because of the high demands of an elderly population, the management of both the acute and the chronically ill in their own homes, new problems of chemotherapy and advances in technology.

The challenge to district nurses today is the gaining of expertise to manage problems that were once difficult to treat. District nurses are developing high level skills in such areas as wound care. There has been extensive research conducted in this sphere and new techniques are available which are evidence based and proven to be effective. The implementation of evidence based practice in wound care, for example, has enabled the healing of chronic wounds such as leg ulcers, which for so long were a significant component of many district nurses caseload.

The millennium and beyond

The Board of Health's community nursing service today is comprehensive and targeted to meeting the changing health needs of the island's population. The district nursing service operates over twenty four hours in support of those people confined to their homes.

However, there is no room for complacency. A flexible and responsive service will be required to meet new demands as new health problems emerge.

The elimination of the infectious diseases had increased life expectancy but allowed non infectious conditions such as degenerative disease and coronary heart disease to become major health problems. It is worth concluding this chapter by reflecting on the past and trying to visualise the future.

Care will change because people will live longer and healthier lives. Community nurses will need to respond to changes in society and to patterns of disease as drugs and technology advance. Nursing care in the community will be increasingly needed by those with chronic illness or disability so that they can remain in their own home and enjoy as much independence as possible.

The information revolution will continue. Personal computers are now commonplace and the Internet will continue to stimulate an information explosion, leading to an increasingly well informed public. Patients and their carers will wish to work in partnership with community nurses, rather than remain passive recipients of professional care. The majority of health care will continue to take place outside hospital, in people's homes, and in clinics and surgeries.

Community nurses in the future face both new challenges but with them will be new opportunities.

Chapter Nine

Health in the Occupation

Ken Tough

Bereft by evacuation of most of its younger people in June 1940 the population of Guernsey aged almost overnight. Planning for the War emergency and then the Occupation forced rapid and radical reform of health services. The Occupation saw clear improvements in maternity care but the most significant contribution to health came from States intervention to maximise food production and ensure its fair distribution.

The Fear of War

From 1935 onwards, fear of devastating aerial bombardment dominated war planning in Britain, under the general title of Air Raid Precautions. Prior to the Munich crisis, in September 1938, this had been little more than a paper exercise. In the final week of that month however, war seemed imminent, provoked by German demands to annex parts of Czechoslovakia. High profile precautions were therefore taken, including the digging of trenches in London parks and the distribution of 38 million gas masks to regional centres; poison gas attack from the air being especially feared.

These developments were reflected in Guernsey. On 29th October 1937 the States approved proposals by the Air Raid Precautions Committee, set up in November 1936, to create an "Air Raid Hospital", with an operating theatre, medical staff etc. The St. John Ambulance Brigade would man First Aid and Decontamination Centres in the heavily populated areas of St. Peter Port and St. Sampson's, relocating six huts from the militia encampment at Les Beaucamps for this purpose. Transport for the wounded would use existing ambulances, augmented by tradesmen's vans.

On 30th September, 1938 the British Prime Minister, Neville Chamberlain, returned from Munich, having reached agreement with Hitler, declaring *"I believe it is peace for our time"*. However, rearmament still proceeded apace, and Air Raid Precautions were suddenly given a much greater priority. On 7th October 1938, the States agreed, as a matter of extreme urgency to purchase gas masks for the civilian population.

The Emergency War Hospital

The States had also agreed that in the event of War, the Country Hospital would be evacuated of its normal inmates, and become the Emergency Hospital. An Auxiliary Nursing Service had been set up including women with nursing experience and others under training. It was pointed out that the required expenditure on beds and other equipment would provide facilities equally valuable in peace or in war, and would be required in any event either by existing hospitals or by the future Island Hospital Service which was being planned.

Within 24 hours of the outbreak of War in September 1939, the Country Hospital was taken over, under an Order signed by the Lieutenant-Governor under the *Emergency War Regulations (Guernsey)* 1939. Patients and inmates were transferred, and by 8th September 1939, the Country Hospital, (now designated the Emergency War Hospital), had been equipped with 190 beds, and was ready to receive patients.

First aid posts and improvised ambulances

The original emphasis in the Air Raid Precautions organisation, of which the Emergency Hospital formed an integral part, was on coping with mass poison gas attacks. An island wide network of 462 Air Raid Wardens, with four First Aid Posts with special provision for gas decontamination had been set up, with minor First Aid Posts in the country areas. Twenty five Mobile First Aid Parties, each of 4 trained personnel in a motorcar with medical equipment, and Ambulances consisting of a lorry with stretcher bearers and equipment, were based at the First Aid Posts. Medical training was supervised by Dr. W. B. Fox, with voluntary assistance from other doctors. The Fire Brigade had been augmented by an Auxiliary Fire Service. The Brigade itself was converted from a part time to full time basis on the outbreak of War.

By November 1939 it was realised that the danger of poison gas attack had been over emphasised and that greater attention should be paid to the risk of incendiary bombs and high explosives. A Heavy and a Light Demolition Party with 36 personnel was organised by the States Engineer, equipped with heavy jacks and housebreaking tools to rescue casualties from collapsed buildings. Master builders H. H. G. Robilliard and G. S. Robilliard in St. Peter Port, Huelins in St. Sampson's, G. Duquemin in the Vale and J. & S. Rabey in St. Martin's, organised Auxiliary Rescue Parties from among their own employees to deal with minor building collapses. The water, gas and electricity utilities set up repair gangs.

The overall Air Raid Precautions organisation had, by November 1939, grown to 1657 volunteer personnel, of which 538 were assigned to First Aid Posts and 203 manned the First Aid Parties and Ambulances. This placed a heavy burden on the training staff, and especially on the instructors of the St. John Ambulance Brigade, at first under Captain Steele and then under J. W. Dear.

A substantial force had therefore been mobilised which would, in the event of a heavy air attack, have channelled a mass of casualties towards the Emergency Hospital, in addition to other wounded who could be expected to make their own way to the Hospital. Would the staff, facilities and organisation of the Emergency Hospital prove equal to the task of coping with air raids and providing general health care for the people of Guernsey?

The German air raid in June, 1940

The initial test came with the German air raid on St. Peter Port Harbour on the early evening of Friday 28th June 1940. This was aimed at what the Germans believed to be a column of military vehicles. In fact, the lorries at St. Peter Port were laden with tomatoes for export to England. In an attack lasting under one hour, 33 civilians were killed, and 35 seriously wounded. The ambulance and police services were in the thick of it; a St. John ambulance was hit and put out of action, and a passing coal lorry had to be used to take the injured to the Emergency Hospital. Overall, the system for dealing with large numbers of casualties worked well, with all available medical and nursing personnel being concentrated in one building, although there was some initial confusion with wounded being taken to the nearby Town Hospital for treatment, instead of to the Emergency Hospital which was at a safe distance from centres of population and likely air targets such as the harbours.

The evacuation of Guernsey schools to the United Kingdom was not planned before the War; it was a decision made by the Guernsey authorities on the 19th June 1940, and the evacuation was completed just two days later. It was fortunate indeed that the raid had not occurred a week later, when the harbour would have been crowded with thousands of school children and adult civilians waiting for the evacuation ships. Two days after the raid the Island was occupied by the Germans.

The Controlling Committee regime

Up until the late spring of 1940, the government of the Island had continued virtually in its peacetime pattern, with frequent States meetings at which all major policy decisions were taken. It was not until the last two weeks of June, in the chaos following the Dunkirk evacuation and the general collapse of the French armies, that the speed of events made change inevitable. The revolutionary process by which the States delegated power to a small 'cabinet' began on 21st June 1940 and was almost complete when the German invasion took place ten days later.

A few finishing touches remained to be added but essentially the pattern of civilian government for the next five years had been established by the end of June, before the Occupation began. States members were summoned by telephone to an emergency meeting at the Royal Court House on Friday, 21st June. They were addressed by Jurat Leale, President of the States Finance Committee, who outlined a new form of government to cope with the emergency.

It was self-evident that the Island would have to submit peacefully to occupation *"The military have gone, we are civilians"* he said. In the present circumstances it was unthinkable to delay decisions for three days, the normal minimum notice for convening a States meeting. Leale explained quite bluntly that *"it must be realised that as at present constituted our system does not work .... The only way out I know is to appoint a small Executive Committee with very large executive powers"*.

After a brief debate of under two hours the States approved the proposals and the Controlling Committee was created, with Ambrose Sherwill, H. M. Procureur, as its first President. The new Committee was given the right to carry out all administrative acts within the power of the States, whether or not contrary to any decision already taken by the States or any existing Committee, whenever such acts appeared to the Committee to require early decision. Its authority was further strengthened on the following day, the 22nd June, when the Royal Court, in exercise of its powers under the *Emergency Powers (Guernsey Defence) Order, 1939* empowered the Committee to control the storage and distribution of articles of any description and to regulate the work of any essential undertaking whenever such action might appear to the Committee *"necessary for maintaining supplies and services essential to the life of the community"*.

Analogous powers were later extended to the Committee for the Control of Essential Commodities by similar means. The States further gave the Controlling Committee full power to pledge the credit of the States to any extent, and to draw on the States Treasurer for its financial requirements. The President was given the right to nominate all the other members of the Committee and, subject to the approval of the Bailiff as President of the States, to remove them. The quorum was to be the President and one other member, or three ordinary members. Thus the Controlling Committee, and its President, were given extraordinary powers far beyond those of peace time committees. Like those committees, it was however ultimately responsible to the States.

The States met infrequently during the Occupation and virtually all significant decisions were made, and implemented, by the Controlling Committee and its members. At a stroke, the traditional method of administration through numerous standing committees, each elected by and responsible to the States for finance, public health, poor law, highways, harbours etc, was replaced by, in effect, a small war cabinet, with each member having his own area of executive responsibilities. The original portfolios were Essential Commodities, Finance and Economics, Agriculture, Horticulture, Labour and Unemployment, Information and Health Services.

Dr. Symons and hospital reorganisation

Dr. Angelo Symons, President of the Board of Health under the peace time regime, was appointed Health Services Officer on the Controlling Committee. He soon exercised the unprecedented powers available to him to re-organise the hospital services, and in particular the management of the Country Hospital.

On the 6th August 1940, Dr. Symons reported to the Controlling Committee on complaints by patients of insufficient food and unsatisfactory conditions generally at the Country Hospital, which had functioned since the outbreak of War as the Island Emergency Hospital, but remained under the control of the States Hospital Board, part of the Public Assistance Authority, which also ran the Town Hospital, and administered outdoor relief to the needy.

Dr. Symons said that the hospital was still being run on workhouse lines. Using the extraordinary powers given to it by the States, the Controlling Committee authorised Dr. Symons to tackle the problems immediately by giving directions as to the diets of patients and staff at the hospital; in addition he was given power to give such directions as he saw fit as regards the management of the medical and nursing departments of the hospital. By any standards this was a sweeping intervention, effectively ousting the Hospital Board from the running of the Country Hospital. It was followed up with a report to the States by Dr. Symons in November 1940. This was brought in his capacity as Health Services Officer rather than as president of a committee, and illustrated how the 'cabinet' style of government through the Controlling Committee had replaced the peace time committees as a means of dealing with the urgent need for swift executive decision and action under enemy occupation.

In his report to the States, Dr. Symons described how, by the end of October 1940, the Island Health Services had been transformed. The Emergency Hospital had become the sole Island Hospital, treating patients of all classes, rich or poor, for surgical or medical care. The patients were treated by doctors of their choice. The Hospital had absorbed the patients and staff of both the Victoria Hospital and the Lady Ozanne Maternity Home when these closed. Some private nursing homes had also closed. The Town Hospital catered for the chronic infirm. The success of this centralisation had been proved by the response to the air raid on the 28th June. All medical and nursing skills were concentrated in the one building and made it easier to deal with the flow of casualties. It minimised the effect of the loss by evacuation of several medical men.

Only nine doctors remained in private practice in Guernsey after the evacuation, together with the Medical Officer of Health and the Medical Superintendant, Mental Health Services, who was later in 1942 to be deported to Germany. One doctor had volunteered to sleep at the hospital each night during the Occupation, and as a result of this public spirited action, the patients had the benefit of a competent medical man on hand, without the difficulties of night-time travel across the Island.

It was agreed by the States that all connections with the workhouse tradition of the former Country Hospital be severed. Patients would pay fees according to their means, with the poor having their fees met from public funds. It was formally renamed the "Emergency Hospital" and was to be run by a new committee of the States. The President and six members were to be elected by the States; and to ensure direct links with the voluntary sector and the medical profession, four additional members were to be appointed, one each by the Victoria Hospital and the Lady Ozanne Maternity Home and two by the local branch of the British Medical Association.

This arrangement would continue for the duration of the War. Dr. Symons proposed that *"the first serious expense after the return to normal will be the provision of a Hospital worthy of modern thought"* Clearly it was recognised that the Emergency Hospital was far more than a response to the immediate crisis of War and Occupation but was also the first step towards a proper general hospital, the full realisation of which would have to await the return of peace.

Revolution in Maternity Care

One unexpected result of the emergency reorganisation of hospital and health provision during the Occupation was a revolution in maternity care. Before the War most births took place at home (60% in 1939); in 1941 the proportion of home confinements fell to 12%, and it never exceeded 18% throughout the Occupation. The switch to hospital or nursing home deliveries was encouraged by health professionals, not just on the grounds of the facilities that the institutions could provide, but also because of the difficulty of travel after curfew, and severe petrol restrictions.

In his report for 1941 the Medical Officer of Health noted that for a second year in succession there had been no deaths in childbirth; the rate of still births was halved during these years and the death rate of infants in the first year of life also showed a reduction on the pre-war experience. This may have been due to a combination of better access to health care and official intervention by rationing; for example, expectant and nursing mothers, and children up to 14 years of age, had a special ration of 1 to 2 pints of whole milk, whereas adults generally were limited to half a pint of separated milk each day.

The Ambulance Service

Integration of Island health services took a further step in December 1939 when the States accepted an offer from the St. John Ambulance Brigade to carry out the whole of the ambulance transport for the Island, with the exception of infectious cases, which were the responsibility of the Board of Health. In return the States agreed to transfer to the Brigade the States ambulance currently operated by the Public Assistance Authority, to provide a new ambulance as and when required, and to provide an annual grant of £200. (Total annual expenditure was estimated at £495, of which the wages of the two employees, a driver and an attendant, accounted for £286).

This approach had been initiated by Dr. W. B. Fox, County Surgeon of the Brigade, and had been brought about by the financial strain of wartime conditions. The Guernsey Division had been formed in 1934; it had two ambulances, one a gift from Jurat John Roussel, the other bought by public subscription. Apart from the two employees, it relied on trained volunteers; the demand on the service had grown, and expenses had now outstripped income from fees and subscriptions. The Public Assistance Authority also operated an ambulance, but was reluctant to transfer this facility to a non States organisation. The States overruled that objection.

The brigade was heavily engaged during the evacuation in June, 1940, transferring invalids from their homes, nursing homes and hospitals to St. Peter Port Harbour. The demands on the service grew after the Occupation began, when private cars were taken off the road for all but the most essential drivers. Ambulances had permits to travel at night, but this was hazardous, because of the blackout and the many German roadblocks manned by nervous and heavily armed sentries. In July, 1940 Dr. Symons strongly advised all expectant mothers to seek prior admission to the Emergency Hospital for their confinement, and warned that any who remained at home did so at their own risk *"as doctors and nurses may not attend during hours of darkness"*. Some mothers did not heed this warning, and added to the nocturnal workload of the ambulance service. Four men, including the Transport Officer Reginald Blanchford, were on permanent duty, and were liable to be called out at any time of the day or night. In February 1941 the States agreed to increase the annual grant to £575 a year.

Maintenance of the fleet of ambulances required ingenuity, for example in obtaining fuel beyond the inadequate ration and in setting up a wind powered generator at the Ambulance Station to enable vehicle batteries to be recharged. Shortage of petrol led to experiments with charcoal powered - gasogene - ambulances and finally, at the end of 1944, with horse-drawn ambulances. An experiment in converting a motor ambulance to horse traction failed - it was too heavy to be drawn by the half-starved horses. A horse-drawn ambulance was then custom built by Mallett's Coachworks, and used from 6th December 1944 onwards. (It served as Sark's ambulance after the War, and is now to be seen at the German Occupation Museum). At the conclusion of the Occupation the ambulance service, under Blanchford's leadership, could claim that no call had gone unanswered, and no patient had died through lack of attendance in an emergency.

Trends in Public Health - Infectious Disease and Sanitation

The Board of Health's primary function at this period was to combat infectious diseases and to monitor trends in public health generally. At the beginning of the Occupation, responsibility for hospital care was fragmented, with the Board of Health, the Hospital Board (part of the poor law system) and voluntary bodies running an uncoordinated range of institutions. The services under the Board's control were, in descending order of expenditure, the Isolation Hospital (King Edward Sanatorium), the Medical Officer of Health and Sanitary Inspectors, the Disinfection Service, the Thalassol Plant (which produced disinfectant from seawater) and the Venereal Diseases Clinic. Dr. Rowan Revell was Medical Officer of Health and Medical Superintendent of the Isolation Hospital; the Venereal Diseases Clinic was run by Dr. Cambridge. The Board of Health itself only met twice during the Occupation, but its President, Dr. Symons, was of course Health Services Officer from June 1940 onwards, with very wide executive powers over all health matters, not just those limited functions of the Board.

From the start of the Occupation, Dr Revell was greatly concerned at the risk of epidemics, especially of such diseases as typhoid, dysentery and typhus. Although the civilian population had been almost halved by the evacuation of June 1940, there had been an almost equivalent influx of German troops, and of foreign workers impressed into service by the Organisation Todt ("OT") to build fortifications. As a result, there was overcrowding in parts of the Town and also in country areas where there was no pre-existing sanitation. Improvised facilities often led to pollution of streams used by the States Water Board. Several cases of typhoid occurred during 1941, three involving civilians, and one of the latter, a nurse, died at the Emergency Hospital.

Tuberculosis, a familiar scourge during the first half of this century, continued to be a killer. Throughout the Occupation pulmonary tuberculosis accounted for the vast majority of admissions to the Isolation Hospital, rising to a peak of 27 deaths in 1944.

Diphtheria inoculation had to be suspended in 1941 for want of reliable vaccines. However, there were no epidemics of childhood diseases during the Occupation, probably because 75% of schoolchildren had been evacuated in 1940 and the improvised war-time schools were very small, often set up in empty houses within easy walking distance of children's homes.

There was very great fear of an outbreak of typhus; this lethal disease was spread by lice that flourished in cold weather in the overcrowded camps and tenements, which were all too common. In the winter of 1941-42 when the Garrison and OT workforce was being reinforced from France where typhus was known to be present, Dr. Revell urged the German authorities to de-louse all persons, both troops and foreign workers, at the ports of embarkation, as the best method of control. The German response was that this was not possible but that measures would be taken for de-lousing after arrival in the Island.

In the event, one outbreak of typhus is known to have occurred in Guernsey. This was in February 1943 and is believed to have been confined to foreign workers of the OT billeted in empty houses in the George Street/Allez Street area of St. Peter Port. The Germans took action to prevent its spread, confining the workers to their dwellings, many of which had become very squalid. No press publicity was given to the outbreak, but organisers of dances were ordered to cancel their events for the next month *"due to unforeseen circumstances"*. Dr. Revell was given no exact information on the outbreak, but he heard that there had been 25 deaths.

The Venereal Diseases Clinic, set up by the Board of Health in 1937, saw a large increase in attendances during the Occupation, with a peak of 2,724 in 1943, 10% for syphilis and 90% for gonorrhoea. Female venereal disease cases were originally isolated in the Town Hospital, but by March 1943 a separate hostel had to be set up in a large, unoccupied house in Hauteville, which was swiftly equipped to take 15 patients. During 1943 a total of 24 cases were admitted.

The Germans required the Clinic to treat French prostitutes imported to serve the garrison; there was indignation when they further directed that the brothel inmates be granted civilian rations at the special rate applicable to workers undertaking exhausting manual work.

Sharing the necessities of life

Before the Occupation, rationing had operated in Guernsey along broadly similar lines to the United Kingdom. The German invasion cut off existing sources of supply and created many difficulties, which had to be coped with without outside assistance or advice. Imports were essential, but could now only be obtained from occupied France; supplies were unpredictable, and often delayed. Production of food in Guernsey was hindered by German requisitioning of land for minefields, fortifications and pasturage of their own horses and other livestock, by unreasonable curfew restrictions shortening the working day, by restrictions on water, gas and electricity, by shortage of fertilisers, by German requisitioning of civilian foodstuffs, by fuel restrictions and by impaired vitality, through under-nourishment, of the whole population.

The civilian population owed its survival to the States-run system of food supply and rationing, augmented from Christmas 1944 by Red Cross relief supplies. The health of the people probably owed more to the equitable distribution of such food and fuel as was available, together with price controls, than to the formal health services. Some enforced dietary changes may have been beneficial, such as the lack of sweets, a reduction in surplus fats and the replacement of white by wholemeal flour. The rations of course fluctuated, and certainly it would have been impossible for anyone to survive on the rationed food alone. The effect of malnutrition was most severe among the elderly, and among Town dwellers with no access to gardens or allotments. The better off could also supplement the ration by purchases of uncontrolled foodstuffs and by recourse to the black market. People generally were of course far less dependent on mains services, such as gas, water and electricity, and better able to shift for themselves, than their descendants in 1999.

Health during the Occupation - an overview

Two contrasting trends can be traced during the Occupation years. Health care could only be maintained at a basic level given the shortage of trained staff, especially medical men, of drugs and equipment. Even diptheria inoculation had to be halted for lack of reliable vaccine. The civilian population, like the physical infrastructure, became more and more run down, and vulnerable groups, especially the elderly or infirm, fell victim to outright malnutrition. There are reports of civilians and even German troops, collapsing in the street from malnutrition and exhaustion in the final months of the Occupation. Infectious diseases were however remarkable by their absence; and fears of typhus or typhoid proved largely unfounded, despite falling standards of sanitation.

The War and the Occupation forced radical changes in the way that health care was provided, with the States intervening to provide a public general hospital to replace the old haphazard range of poor law and voluntary institutions.

As with the Emergency Medical Service in England, from which developed the National Health Service, the Guernsey Emergency Hospital paved the way for the post-war general hospital run by the States. It was ironic that the Germans should have been the first to recognise the potential of the brand new Mental Hospital at Le Vauquiedor by ousting the patients in 1941 and converting it to become their military general hospital. That conversion became permanent when in 1949 the Princess Elizabeth Hospital was opened in the buildings at Le Vauquiedor. The mental patients were rehoused in the Country Hospital where they were to remain for the next fifty years.

Other significant advances were made in maternity care, when hospital deliveries became the norm rather than the exception, and in the integration of ambulance provision under the St. John Ambulance Brigade. Some positive results therefore emerged from the trauma of German Occupation.

Main sources

Billets d'Etat of the States of Guernsey: 1936-1946

Channel Islands Occupation Birth Cohort Study (in progress -personal communication from Dr George Ellison, Department of Biological Anthropology, Cambridge)

Channel Islands Occupation Review: Guernsey & Jersey 1973 - ongoing

Controlling Committee minutes: 1940-1945 (Island Archives)

Wood, Alan & Mary: Islands in Danger: London, 1955

97

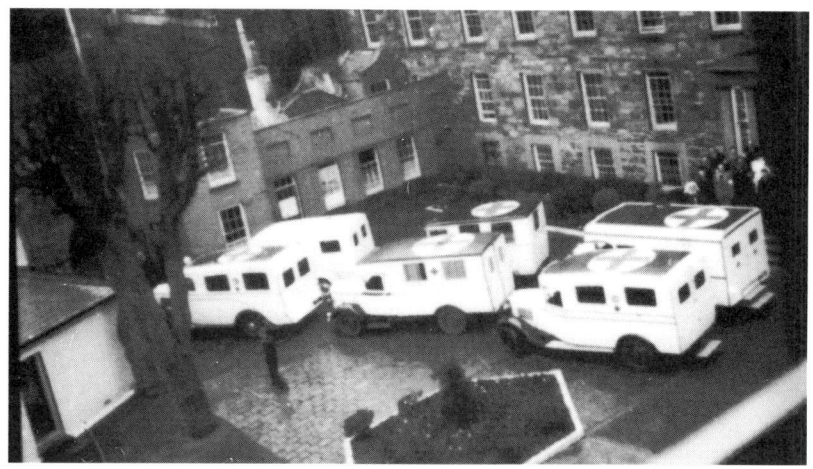

'On 25th and 26th March 1943 the Town Hospital was evacuated whilst the German's had artillery practice' (Chapter Three)

Especially built horse drawn ambulance used by St John during the Occupation. It was made by coach builders Malletts. (Chapter Nine)

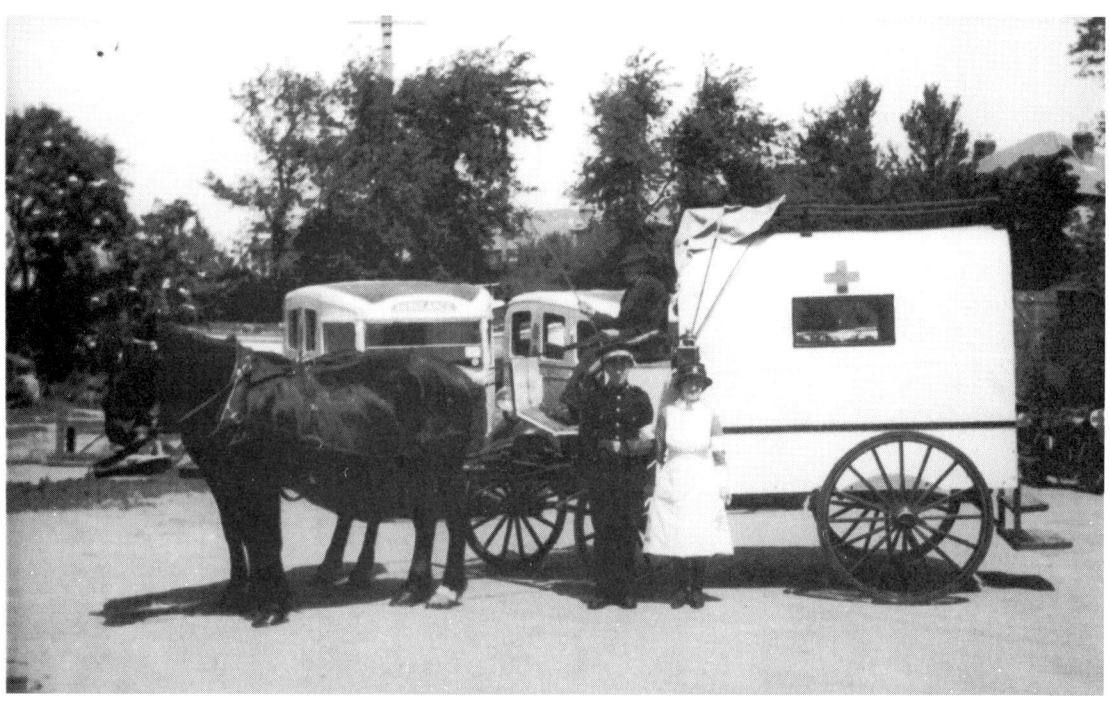

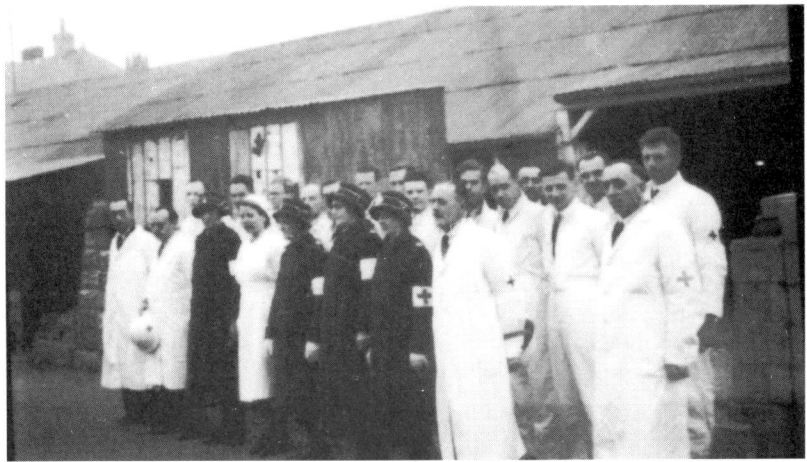

A group of St John personnel pictures during the Occupation, the men in white coats and boiler suits because the Germans initially forbade the wearing of any uniforms. (Chapter Fourteen)

Another sick islander leaves home on a stretcher. Poor nutrition was the main cause of a drastic drop in the population's health. (Chapter Nine)

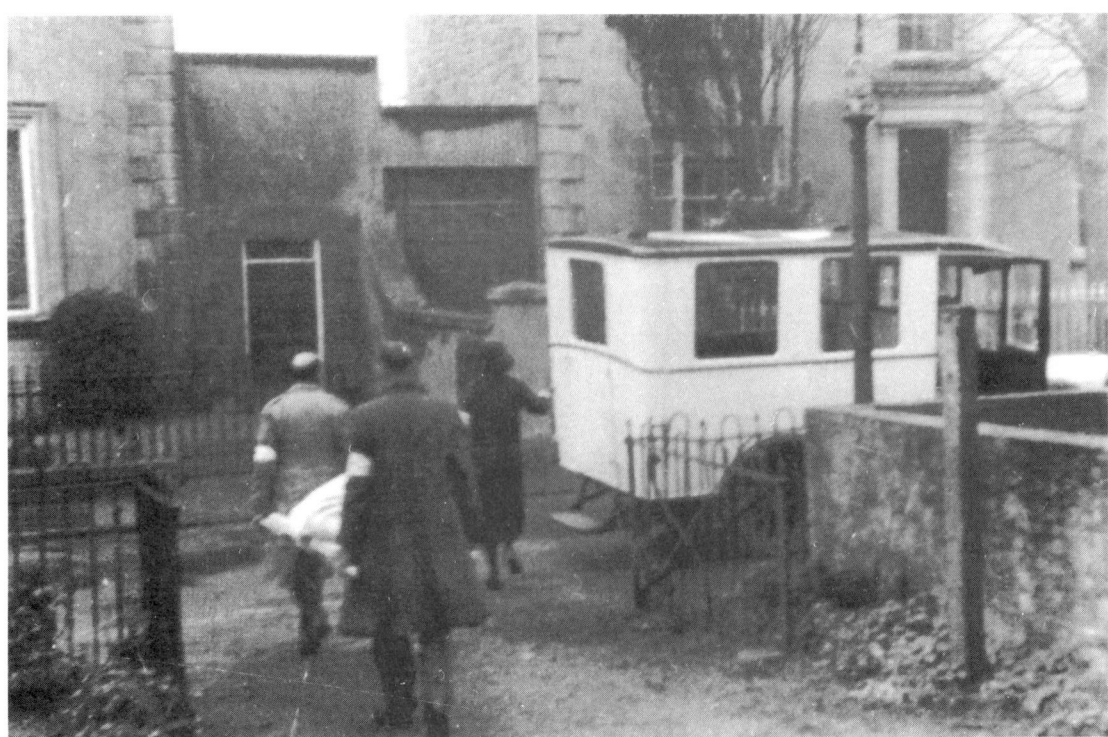

Chapter Ten

The post-war period

Dr Brian Seth-Smith

While the National Health Service was being established in Britain, Guernsey chose to follow a different course. The growth of group practice, with 'generalists' and 'specialists' working alongside one another became the established pattern. Several local doctors recall experiences in a system which was unusual in Europe, although more common in countries such as Australia and Canada.

After the Occupation

This review of medical practice covers the post-war years, when medical care provided by group practices flourished until the 'big bang' of 1991 with the resulting formation of a separate Medical Specialist Group. Such a long period allows only somewhat superficial coverage of the changes during that time - nevertheless, it gives an impression, if a somewhat personal one, of the many changes in health care during those years.

Sadly, the early post-war period has become somewhat indistinct, since none of the doctors who experienced the German occupation remain with us. How one wishes one could have sat with the likes of Dr. Bill Fox, Dr Alastair Rose, or Dr. Brook Sutcliffe to record some of their wonderful anecdotes of medical practice during that period. Readers who were here then will, I am sure be able to recall tales of medical ingenuity, and resulting successes and failures from those years.

The group practice system that developed in Guernsey differed fundamentally from that on the mainland for two main reasons. Firstly, our general hospital did not have its own staff, and was from the beginning run by the general practitioners. In addition, because of our relative isolation, we needed medical facilities of a far more comprehensive range than an equivalent mainland cottage hospital.

Outside help was not available in emergency situations, and as a result there was a tradition of recruiting doctors with special interests and skills. The pattern had been started by the largest group in St. Sampson's, who already carried a qualified surgeon and who had then recruited Dr Heyworth in 1937 into a post advertised for *"a general practitioner specialising in anaesthetics."* During the post-war period many new doctors who might, be described as "semispecialists" came here because they were attracted by the combination of being able to provide personal medical care with the practice of their special interest in the hospital.

Medical care in the island therefore tended to be given by doctors "wearing two hats", and there was within the profession a remarkable aversion to those who described themselves as specialists. A good example was the custom for surgeons to abandon the use of their appellation 'Mr', which was customary in Britain, and to return to being known as 'Doctor' - thus abandoning any claim to special status. Indeed one surgeon who styled himself 'Mr' was thought by others to have been advertising! This curious custom does however emphasise the great camaraderie amongst the majority of doctors in the early post war period.

Whilst the encouragement of 'specialism' within general practice produced high quality personal and hospital care, particularly in terms of good liaison with patients during their illnesses, it contained the antecedents of its own destruction.

Doctors began to find it increasingly difficult to maintain really high technical standards of hospital specialist work whilst still undertaking general practice consultations and offering the home visits which patients still demanded. Thus surgeons, with one notable exception, began to give up general practice and were later succeeded by younger surgeons who had no intention of practising as generalists at all. Other specialisms, such as anaesthetics, also came under increasing demand in order to support their surgical colleagues.

Internal tensions within practices therefore developed due to the difficulties of organising fair and equitable on-call rotas, whilst still providing hospital cover at all times.

Throughout the post-war years, the rate of change, particularly in hospital medicine, became more rapid, whilst each group tried to recruit the type of specialists they considered most needed in order that their groups could offer as comprehensive a service as possible. The competitive aspect of this began to threaten the balance of available specialists and the need for overall planning for the island's health needs began to replace the previous uncontrolled developments of individual practices. The scene was set for separate planning of specialist services for the island as a whole.

Despite all these difficulties and disadvantages, the system served Guernsey well up until the end, perhaps because of the excellent co-operation that had grown between the six groups of doctors. By 1990 the hospital specialist rotas were well established.

Writing of this period, Dr Jim Dickson recalls *'Co-operation between surgeons allowed time off, holidays and the performance of more complicated operations such as the removal of cancer of lower bowel by two surgical teams working together. Annual meetings to order new instruments became weekly meetings to discuss mutual problems, and the introduction of Saturday morning ward rounds for the bedside discussion of patient care, which involved both nurses and physiotherapists proved most valuable'*.

General practitioners too had come to terms with their 'competing' colleagues, and patients had become accustomed to visiting what would at one time have been considered 'rival' surgeries to see whoever was considered the best qualified doctor to deal with a particular problem. Many doctors and patients were sad to see the system change, but the continuing progress in health technology had made change inevitable.

There are some who claim however that this came at a high cost, since many of the personal aspects of medical care have suffered in the separation between general practitioners and specialists. The late Dr Brian Webber sadly recalled *'The end of the round-the-clock doctor, who was family friend, counsellor and provider of personal medical services, which together made for a fulfilling professional career'*.

The early post war years

In 1945 medical care generally remained an "ad hoc" affair. Patients waited until an illness occurred, then called the doctor if really necessary, when they usually arranged a visit from someone they already knew. Although some doctors were already in partnership, they rarely stood in for one another, and most doctors were "on call" all the time. Some were sufficiently relaxed to go on fishing trips and to expect their patients to await their return.

Most of the surgeries were in part of the doctors' own homes, but much more of their time was spent doing home visits than in surgery consultations. Very few, if any, medical notes were written. Doctors relied on their memory and personal knowledge of their patients. As late as the 1960's I recall being impressed with the knowledge held by the older doctors, which must have resulted from the fact that so little had been written.

There was no hospital record system, with the result that details of the work at the Emergency Hospital are anecdotal rather that factual. Most of the medical consultations were private, and by the 1960's consultation fees had risen to 7/6d (or 38p) which always included a bottle of medicine. I remember being gently admonished if I did not provide the bottle, as it was an considered an essential part of the therapeutic process, whatever coloured liquid it contained.

Patients were billed quarterly, and not surprisingly there were a considerable number of unpaid accounts. In those years I believe it was not "done" to take action of these apart from sending repeated reminders. During the Occupation various barter transactions had become accepted, and this also applied to the payment of doctors.

It is well to recall the poor health of the Islanders at the end of the war. Dr A N Symons, the Medical Officer on the Controlling Committee throughout the war described the situation graphically. There were various calculations of the average calorie intake of the citizens, but it had probably dropped to below 2000 calories. Most had suffered weight loss, and general lethargy was widespread. Tuberculosis was not uncommon, and cases of diphtheria also occurred. Nevertheless the majority regained their health quite rapidly, and much was done in the first year of Liberation to restore their diet with the help of nutritionists on the mainland.

The work of Dr A N Symons during the post-war years needs special mention. He was a New Zealander who had practised in Jersey for many years before coming to Guernsey to retire. However, by the time war came he had served as a Douzenier, was on 21 States Committees, and had been elected as President of the Board of Health in 1939. It is little wonder that at the outset of the Occupation period, he was asked to serve as the Medical Officer of the Controlling Committee, which virtually ran the island under the watchful eye of the Germans, and his contribution to the maintenance of health amongst the citizens in times of great hardship was incalculable. He continued as President of the Board of Health until the end of 1948.

Whilst the Board of Health was beginning to take a more strategic view of the health needs of the island, the 14 or so general practitioners were increasingly inter dependent, particularly when surgical treatment became necessary. Nevertheless, there were many practitioners still doing operations themselves, often kindly assisted and advised by Dr 'Dick' Gibson who was a Fellow of the Royal College of Surgeons (FRCS).

Despite this and many other examples of friendship between doctors, inflexible and paternalistic attitudes prevented full co-operation. It took many years to eradicate the once common idea that to see another doctor's patient was unprofessional. Indeed there were complaints to the Board about delays in the Receiving Room (formed much later on), despite a doctor being on the premises from another practice. Of course, rotas were gradually introduced as the system opened up, whilst it has to be said that not all doctors shared these rather rigid attitudes.

The concept of having one general hospital for the Island had now been fully accepted. Any doctor who had passed through the routine of appearing before Royal Court for permission to practice appears to have been accepted to treat their patients at the Emergency Hospital. Some of the general practitioners were competent general surgeons, but the great majority of operations were performed by Dr 'Dick' Gibson. He had joined in partnership with his uncle in 1919 after very distinguished service in the RAMC., and had later qualified FRCS He had remained in the Island during the Occupation and had performed most of the operative surgery throughout that period. He continued as the only Fellow of the Royal College of Surgeons for some years until his retirement. He was a distinguished island citizen, and became a Jurat of the Royal Court. His wartime colleague, Dr R B ("Brook") Sutcliffe, was later awarded a similar distinction.

The general hospital (as the Castel 'Emergency Hospital' had become) began to be the place for doctors to meet and discuss problems, so that at the time of my arrival in 1960 the PEH had become central to our daily work. Most doctors had patients in the hospital, and always called to obtain their mail and 'Path Lab' or 'X-ray' reports. Even if their patients had, for instance, been treated by specialist surgeons, the GP was still expected to look after their day-to-day care.

Dr. J E T Strickland lists some 15 doctors working here at the time of his appointment in 1947. Ten years later there were six fully established practices, and by then only members of those practices could use the facilities of the hospitals.

The late Dr Brian Webber has written *'Being supernumerary, I was denied the privilege accorded to every other GP of being appointed to the medical staff of the hospital. However, I was allowed to treat patients in the hospital under the supervision of my two partners, although deprived of the privilege of admitting and, discharging patients. In the event this proved to be no hindrance, as I simply had to say to the Matron or Night Sister 'I am deputising for my partner, whose patient needs admission'. In fact there was a brief period when I found myself in sole charge of more than half the patients in the female medical ward'.*

The facilities at the Emergency Hospital were fairly basic. It had no laboratory or X ray department, and I believe the toilet facilities in the wards were grossly inadequate, although this was perhaps alleviated by the fact that most patients were kept in bed throughout their stay! A section of the hospital continued to be used for maternity patients, and it was not until 1948 that the Victoria Hospital at Amherst was opened as the Maternity Home. All the post-war practitioners were expected to perform midwifery, only some of whom had had special training, and these were called in to assist with any complications.

Whilst Amherst was popular with patients, nurses and doctors, it suffered greatly by the absence of operating facilities. Patients needing a planned Caesarean Section, and those who were thought to be at some risk of perhaps requiring one in an emergency were treated in a ward converted for that purpose at the PEH, but there remained a number of unfortunate women who had to be transferred by ambulance in distressing circumstances. This situation persisted over many years despite several recommendations for all maternity cases to be treated in a planned maternity ward at the PEH.

The origins of the Princess Elizabeth Hospital

There is little evidence in the pre-war years of moves to improve hospital conditions apart from those for the mentally retarded and the mentally ill. There had however been a long term call to combine the facilities at the Town and Country hospitals, and the "Lady Ozanne Maternity Home" into one General hospital, possessing a laboratory, and X-Ray Department, and wards for 250 patients, together with arrangements for a resident doctor! A Hospital Investigation Committee was formed, which confirmed the principle of having the single institution, but no site was found, and no progress had been made by 1939.

The needs of the Mental Health Committee must have been thought greater, and what was then called the Vauquiedor Hospital had been built for their use on land described as a *'beautiful wooded estate'*, which had been sold to the States. The building was never used for its intended purpose, being partly taken over by the Germans as a military hospital in 1940.

It must have been a bitter disappointment to the then psychiatrist, Dr McGlashan, who had been the driving force behind the setting up of a *"modern Mental Hospital"* to have the building taken from his hands as our General Hospital. However, the Board had received a very unfavourable report on the conditions inside the Castel building, when it was functioning as a general hospital, and this was strongly reinforced by the report of Drs Bourne, Grundy and Beardsall in early 1946.

Thus once again the needs of the mentally ill patients were given lower priority, and indeed they have remained at the Castel Hospital to this day. A mainland architect trained in hospital design Mr Milburn was chosen to design the conversion of the Vauquiedor Hospital into a general hospital, which involved the installation of lifts, wider staircases, a central heating system, etc.

On 26th July 1949 the building was formally opened by the, then Princess Elizabeth. There had been ongoing debates about the proposed name, and there was some support for the *"Guernsey General Hospital"*. However, permission from Buckingham Palace was freely given for the Royal appellation, so the *'Princess Elizabeth Hospital'* it became. Pathology was catered for in a basic fashion and two rooms were converted as operating theatres, one for minor surgery and one as a main theatre. At that time there were plans for a modern 'Operating Suite" with separate "scrub" facilities etc., but these never materialised. In fact the theatres there served us very well right up to the time of the opening of the present Theatre Block.

For the next 50 years the hospital continually developed. At the beginning the theatres and surgical beds were on the ground floor. The same block held the Children's Ward, which was later converted into the Receiving Room, or Casualty Department. Right up to 1962 we had to treat "casualty" patients in a room off the surgical wards, and some of the more senior doctors were very half-hearted about the prospect of a Department for that purpose!

Radiology

An X-Ray Department was completed and opened in August 1952. The planning for this had been assisted by Dr Alec Orlay, a doctor practising privately from consulting rooms in The Grange. Up till then, patients had had to be transferred there to be x-rayed.

The equipment in the new department included one or two of the German machines left behind by the occupying forces. Dr Jim Dickson recalls *'a small x-ray machine left by the Germans played its part, and the hospital carpenter was asked to make a wooden box to hold the film under the patient. He took it upon himself to smarten it up with a thick coat of Guernsey greenhouse paint. Unfortunately, this was heavily leaded, and was therefore impervious to x-rays. Modifications were needed!!!'*

Dr Symons, who had retired as BoH President some time earlier, was asked to perform the opening ceremony. From the very beginning, the department was used at above expected capacity, and it has never ceased expanding.

The previous month the States had broken new ground by agreeing to appoint a Consultant Radiologist to run the department. Dr John Bulstrode, a graduate of Guy's Hospital who had served in the wartime Navy, was appointed and for a time was the one and only States Consultant. I believe his appointment was not wholeheartedly welcomed by the Finance and Advisory Committee, who soon had to match his salary to the scale equivalent to (but not exactly the same as) that of an NHS Consultant.

Nor were some of the doctors too keen, seeing the beginning of States-appointed doctors in the hospital and fearing for their future livelihood. Many battles were to follow over the matter of Consultant remuneration, but Dr Bulstrode personally became very popular amongst the doctors by giving them a competent, reliable and efficient service.

Pathology

Equally interesting was the early formation of the Pathological Laboratory. Late in 1946 the Board of health had advertised for a Laboratory Technician, and had interviewed a Mr. H A Wilson for the post. Almost immediately he started work, the Board began to receive praise for his work, as Mr. Michael Symons recalls.

"Henry Wilson originally set up a small public Health Laboratory at Lukis House in the Grange. He soon moved to the two small rooms just inside the old main door of the Princess Elizabeth Hospital, long before it was renovated and occupied by anyone else. The only heating was by open coalfire. The laboratory was mainly furnished by equipment that Henry had salvaged from laboratory equipment and supplies left behind by the German occupying forces.

Those early years were marked by rapid growth combined with severe financial constraints. This caused considerable conflict between Henry and some of those in administration, as the legitimate requests for laboratory tests by Medical Staff, Veterinary Staff, and Public Health continually multiplied. I remember his fury when a President of the Board of Health gave instructions that we should write our reports in pencil to save costs of disposable ball-point pens (we continued to use ball point pens)'.

An enormous amount of work was covered by the Laboratory, 50% or so of which was veterinary and public health investigation. Tuberculosis was a major concern as was the need to improve the laboratory conditions to reduce the risks to the staff. A blood transfusion service was set up with the co-operation of some of the doctors who had received training in the subject, and of the St John Ambulance Brigade. The only main branch of pathology which Mr Wilson could not cover was histopathology (the microscopic examination of tissue samples).

These arrangements continued until the appointment of a Consultant Pathologist following an extensive report on Guernsey Medical Services (the Milnes Walker Report) in 1973. By that time Henry Wilson had overseen the steady extension of the laboratory into a modern and efficient department, and both Mr Symons and many of the doctors who knew him feel that his services have not been sufficiently recognised. As Michael says, *"He did not always receive the credit he deserved".*

The new hospital grows

The Board of Health began a "long-term plan" for the development of the new hospital in the 1960's. An architect from England with hospital experience was engaged and new developments were planned in phases. Phase 1A was the construction of a new Children's Ward between two arms of the existing building, and phase 1B was a major plan to include surgical wards, operating theatres, central sterilising department, pharmacy, post-mortem room, and supporting service areas.

The first version of the plan was presented to the States in 1966. The debate, which I attended was animated. One speaker did not wish the inclusion of a mortuary as he could not understand why money should be spent on the dead, whilst the President of the Advisory and Finance Committee thought the overall plans too grandiose. In particular, the use of a "mainland" architect was not popular, and the Board was asked to reconsider the project.

On reflection, I think this was a fortunate decision, as the revised plans, submitted and approved by the States in 1971 were undoubtedly far superior. The States had appointed Mr K Woodhead as their architect, who worked closely with the Planning Committee and others to produce an excellent design which continues to be the central part of the hospital, The local building firm of Gamble and Blair was engaged as the prime contractor. The new design necessitated relocating the main entrance, but left the X-ray Department and the "Receiving Room" (A&E Dept.) at the Vauquiedor end, far from the theatres and surgical wards.

This separation was unsatisfactory in many ways. Minor cases for theatre had to be taken long distances through the hospital and in particular it was difficult to develop a plan to deal with major disasters, the possibility of which was always under consideration.

Despite these disadvantages Phase 1 was widely welcomed and the building was officially opened by the Queen Mother in the summer of 1986. The new wards, divided into four-bedded bays, were popular, and there were few serious problems with the theatres, air conditioning, etc. (though later much asbestos had to be removed!). Active planning of the next phases continued, but is was not until 1991 that the next major change was completed, with the A&E. and X-Ray Departments finally in their proper place, and with planned accommodation for the steadily increasing number of day-stay patients. Sadly, the medical wards have not shared in this progress, and is an outstanding need still to be addressed.

Such continuing developments have also led to a growth in administration. Dr Jim Dickson recalls *'When I came in 1955 there were three offices in the hospital, one for the Secretary, one for the Matron, and one for the Consultant Radiologist. There was car parking for twenty cars, and only about twenty doctors on the staff '.*

Changes in general practice

Practice modernisation included the construction of purpose-built surgeries, later becoming the rather more grandly titled 'Health Centres'. VHF radios began to be used in the 1960s, subsequently replaced by mobile telephones, and these transformed communications within the groups. By 1985, the connections between many general practitioners in their surgeries, and hospital practice became rather distant, so group practices might contain partners whose daily routines varied considerably. Some of the six groups were beginning to consider the advantages of further amalgamation.

Despite the formation of a Medical Staff Committee by the doctors to advise the Board on all hospital matters, it was the composition of the hospital medical staff which most concerned the Board of Health. There seemed to them to be too many doctors, and too little control or regulation. An external report in 1969 recommended the Board consider the appointment of salaried specialists, but this idea was not pursued. Later in 1985, a powerful team headed by Sir Douglas Black arrived *"to review the arrangements for health care in Guernsey and to advise on future development."*

Their extensive report commented *"the established custom of incorporating specialities within what is essentially a general practice framework may have to be reviewed"*. The report concluded there were too many obstetricians and too many physicians, and that surgical recruitment should be better organised. The seeds for change had been sown, the change that was to grow from them is further described in Chapters Twelve and Thirteen.

UK and the Reciprocal Agreement.

The island has always needed outside medical support and continues to do so, despite having increased the range of local facilities. Historically, Guy's Hospital played a major part, mainly due to contacts with their surgeon, Sir Heneage Ogilvie, who attended the 1949 opening ceremony, and to this day patients are still referred there. For the majority, however, mainland referrals tended to go to the Wessex centres of Southampton and Portsmouth.

Another advance was the first introduction of clinics by a mainland consultant in his paid NHS time. These were pioneered by Dr. Peter Bodkin, the Consultant Radiotherapist at the Royal South Hants Hospital, and enabled seriously ill patients to be seen by him both before and after treatment. His successor continues the practice, and other speciality clinics have been added on a similar basis.

Contacts with medical specialists had always been much valued by local doctors. Dr John Strickland recalls *'these consultants would either arrange to admit patients to hospitals in England under their care, or perhaps operate upon them here in Guernsey or just offer them opinions at consultations. They were all extremely helpful and local doctors learned much from their visits. On many occasions they would operate upon patients locally without charging a fee if the doctor suggested it'.*

The passing of the old style Guernsey practice of the post war years was mourned by many, both doctors who were able to practice their skills in hospital and community settings, and by patients who benefited from this very personal level of care.

Despite very grave foreboding of those doctors who opposed the formation of a separate specialist group, the transition passed remarkably smoothly, and I believe that much of the 'stage-setting' for this had been done by the rapidly-changing group practices themselves, during the exciting years I have tried to describe.

Acknowledgements

A number of doctors who were in practice in the post war years have kindly shared reminiscences and anecdotes. Inevitably it has not been possible to include all these, but special acknowledgements are due to Dr Jim Dickson, Dr John Strickland, and the late Dr Brian Webber - Editor.

The post-war period

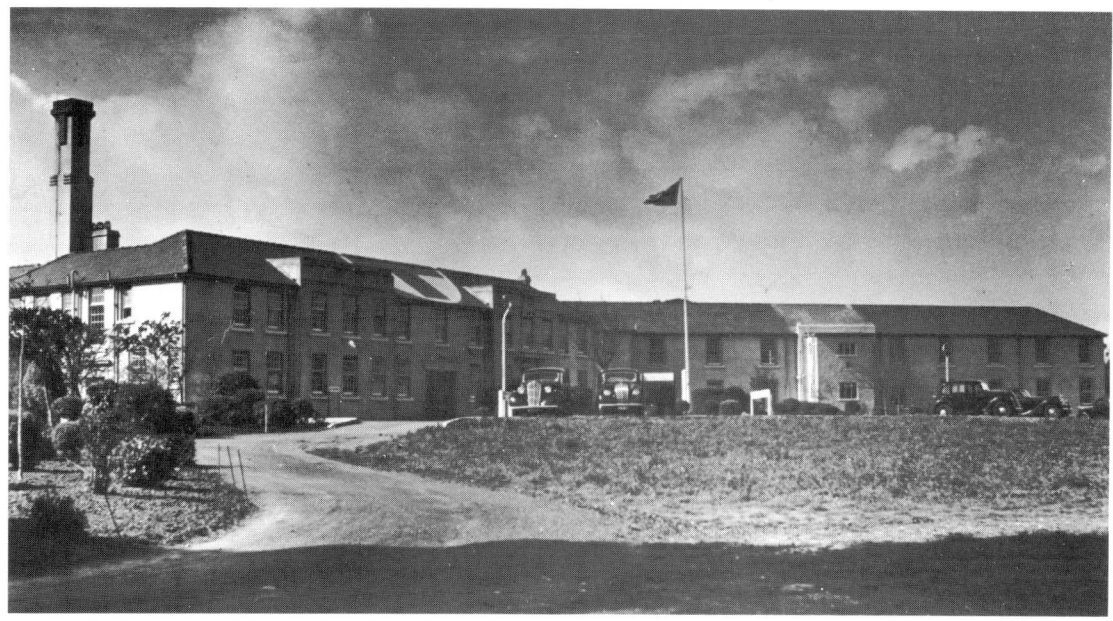

The Vauquiedor Hospital shortly after the Liberation. Note the red cross on the roof - from when it was partially used as a German Military Hospital. (Chapter Ten)

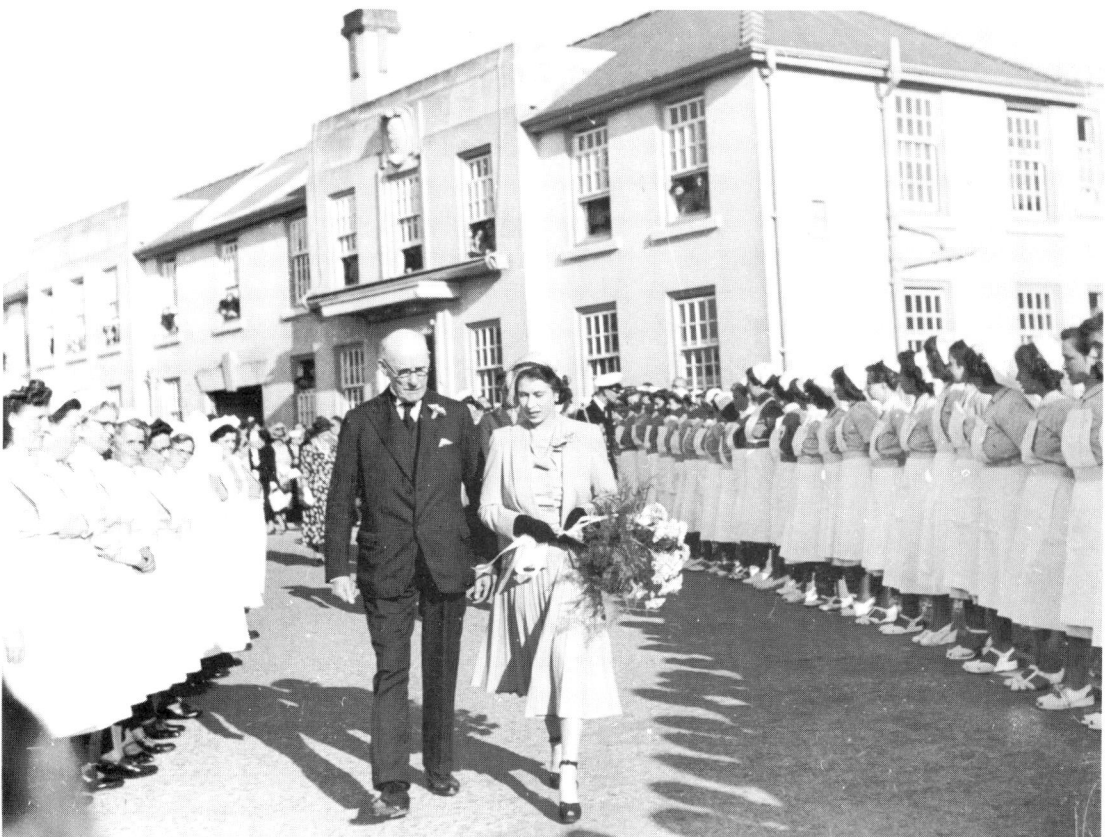

Her Royal Highness The Princess Elizabeth accompanied by Dr A N Symons, President of the Board of Health passes between a guard of honour formed by nurses as she returns to her car on 23rd June 1949. (Chapter Ten)

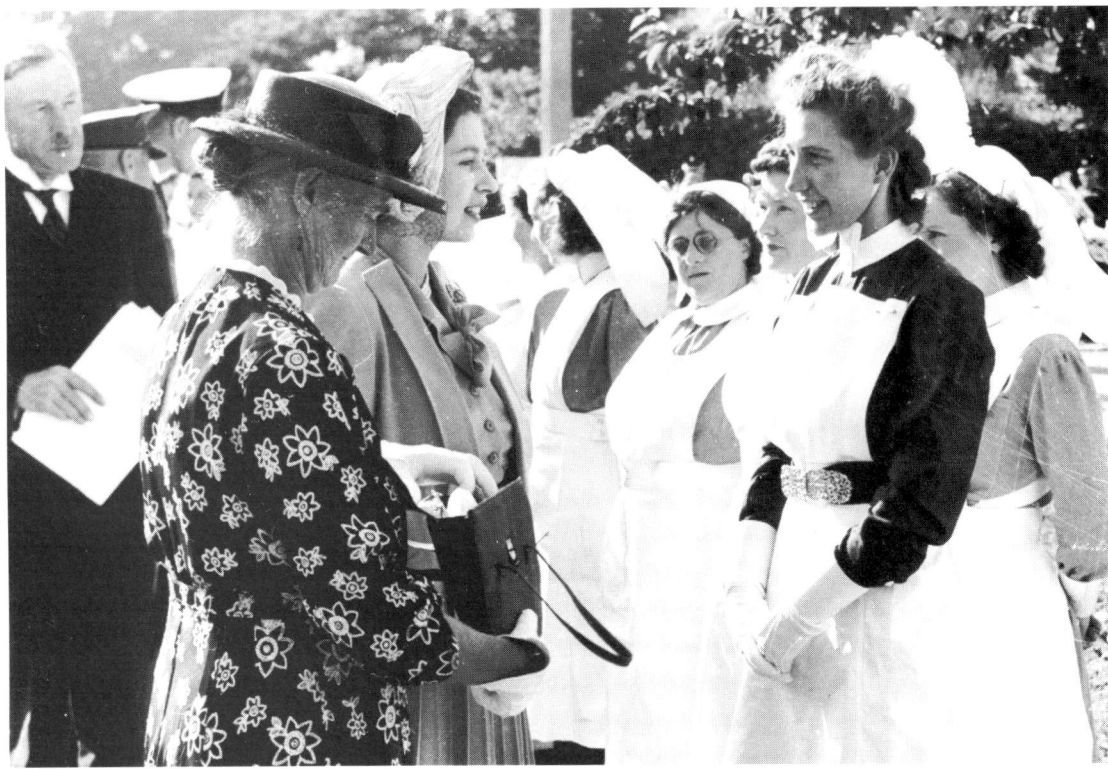
Royal Visits I: Deputy Miss Marie Randall presents Sister C M Bones of the Town Hospital to Her Royal Highness The Princess Elizabeth. (Chapter Ten)

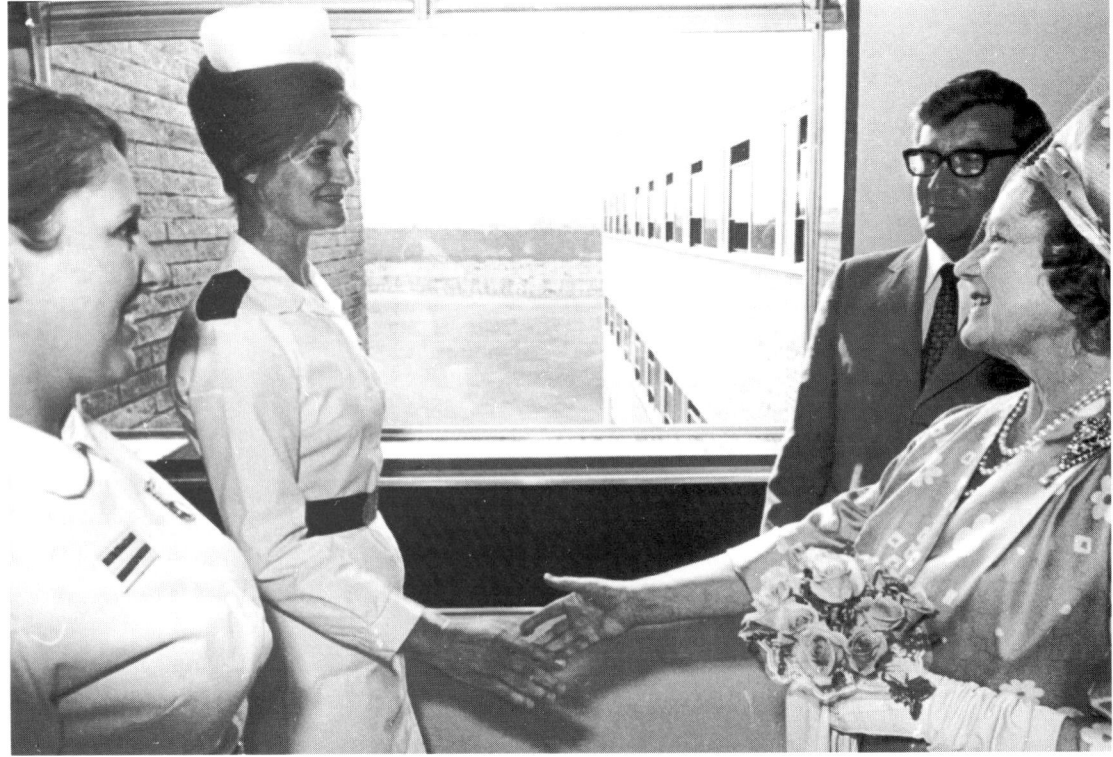
Royal Visits II: Mr P Kelly Nursing Officer presents Sister C Sarre and Sister M H Paul to Her Majesty Queen Elizabeth The Queen Mother 28th May 1975. (Chapter Ten)

Chapter Eleven

Pressures for change - A Specialist View

Mr Roger Allsopp FRCS LLM

Technical advances, increasing specialisation, and rising health care costs together led to tensions within the group practices, and confrontation with States Committees. The medical profession recognised the need for change, but it was political pressure that eventually forced the separation of primary from secondary care, and led to the formation of the Medical Specialist Group. This in turn paved the way for the introduction of the Health Insurance Scheme.

The background to change

In the early post war years, Guernsey decided against emulating the National Health Service in Britain. Doctors remained in private practice, patients paying for the services of their doctor. As the individual doctors built up their practices, they found it difficult to cope with the increase in the quantity and scope of their work, and so appointed assistants and later partners, resulting in the development of group practice.

This chapter deals with the last twenty-five years, 1975 to date, and is concerned with the changes that were brought about by the need for increasing specialisation within these group practices.

Change was brought about by a variety of factors. There was the clinical need for change to keep abreast of technical developments, and the political need to address the increasing costs of providing health care for the Island. Costs were of concern to patients who had to pay for individual medical services, they were of concern to doctors who wished to maintain their financial independence against mounting public criticism of the regular increases in medical fees, and they were of concern to politicians who ultimately had to underwrite the costs of health services.

The years 1985 to 1990 were an unsettled time for the medical profession in Guernsey, with much debate about possible reform. It was a time of independent reviews and great soul searching amongst those responsible for the provision of care. A report by the Board of Health to the States in November 1989, was to mark a turning point in the future planning and funding of health services. From the subsequent debate came the opportunity to radically restructure medical care in Guernsey, specifically with regard to the delivery of specialist services. As a direct consequence came the opportunity to consider compulsory health insurance for these services.

The separation of specialists from group practice in 1992 led perhaps inevitably to the introduction of the Specialist Insurance Scheme which was to follow in 1995.

Group Practice: 1975-1992

The Guernsey system of medical care worked well in 1975. The system was almost unique at a time when large group practices were uncommon in the United Kingdom. Doctors in Guernsey were generally well qualified, with many having a considerable number of postgraduate degrees and diplomas, and specialist interests and skills.

Patients could enrol with any practice that they wished. There were no automatic 'grants', so the practices were in competition with respect to the services they could offer and the prices they could charge. There were no standard fees, the emphasis was on 'value for money'. Reputation was all important, patients learned by word of mouth and made their choice. Doctors for their part "guarded" their patients, and tried to give individual and personal service. The patient for example, registered with a particular doctor, would as a rule see that particular doctor who would care for them and probably their family both in and out of hospital.

The doctor attended or was responsible for their entry into the world, and the doctor was aware of the social circumstances surrounding the family. The families' ability to pay was taken into account when submitting charges. On rare occasions, a system which had been common during the Occupation years persisted, whereby the doctor accepted small gifts of tomatoes, flowers or melons in lieu of fees. The Social Insurance Authority paid the fees of those patients who were genuinely in need, using a system of means testing.

Family doctors were by and large highly regarded in Guernsey society. Many had received private education, and graduated through Oxford, Cambridge and London. Some had come to the Island with private means, most lived well and there was a lack of commercialisation. All this was to change. Up until 1975, the cost of living in Guernsey had been reasonable in comparison with Britain. The 'Thatcher boom' saw a period of high inflation in both the United Kingdom and Guernsey.

Specialist doctors were generally attracted to the Island by the potential for delivering a high standard of care in the excellent facilities offered in the new phase II development at the Princess Elizabeth Hospital. However, they were financially in a very different position from earlier generations of doctors. The average period of training for a specialist was ten years after obtaining a basic medical degree, and these ten years were spent in junior and middle grade hospital appointments. Specialist training was fiercely competitive, involving very long hours of work at very low rates of pay. As a result of their long training, specialists were rarely below the age of thirty-five, and had had little opportunity to accumulate funds whilst working in junior grade posts in the NHS.

Arriving in Guernsey, they found it very difficult to buy houses in a rising market, and at the same time to pay the substantial sums demanded to purchase 'good will' in order to become a full partner in a group practice.

Their situation was compounded by the Housing Authority insisting that doctors coming into the Island buy houses at the top end of the market, resulting in intense financial pressures on incoming specialists.

This was in contrast to those who had opted for a career in general practice, who had generally taken up posts at an earlier age. These financial matters are mentioned because they have importance on understanding the changes that were to occur. Junior doctors in Britain had finally achieved financial improvement by negotiating an 'hourly rate'. When this 'hourly rate' was compared with financial rewards in Guernsey, doctors felt they should charge far more for their services if they were to retain a competitive advantage with their with their mainland colleagues, and so continue to attract specialists in the future.

The need for change

Although doctors remained in private practice, the States of Guernsey were responsible for a proportion of doctors fees. Pay negotiations between doctors, the Board of Health and the States Insurance Authority in the early eighties were often prolonged and acrimonious.

The doctors of a previous generation may have been regarded as 'gentlemen', but they were rarely businessmen. Outstanding fees were usually not pursued with zeal, and the 'Robin Hood' principle sometimes prevailed, where more affluent patients were charged more to make up this shortfall from those who could ill afford to pay.

As a consequence, many doctors felt that their relative financial position was deteriorating, and when faced with a more robust attitude from the States bodies, they began increasingly to employ accountants, legal advisors and to seek the support of the BMA in London. There was a level of confrontation that was new to the Island although doctors fees only represented a small part of the overall health care budget.

However, the increasing technical complexity of medical interventions, and the greater opportunities presented following the opening of Phase II of the PEH, had led to an increase in specialist procedures, which in turn had lead to a greater increase in hospital costs - 75% of which related to staff costs.

Faced with these escalating costs the Board of Health attempted to reach agreement with doctors representatives on possible ways to limit expenditure and develop health care priorities. Many in the profession were of the view however that any patient who sought medical advice and treatment was entitled to receive it, and the doctor was duty bound to provide. The alternative perception was that doctors in private partnerships were running businesses, with a financial incentive to expand their time and work, whilst the Board of Health had a fixed budget with which to try to meet this uncapped demand.

Meanwhile, specialists appointed to a group practice were concerned that they were having to undertake too broad a range of specialist procedures. Although there was a certain amount of interchange of work with other practices, there was also a certain reluctance to refer patients between practices. As time went on, doctors did in fact refer many more patients outside their own practices, but the mechanisms of referral and the financial arrangements were cumbersome.

Of greater concern to the specialists at the time was the perceived lack of planning with respect to the overall medical manpower. Specialists and some general practitioners shared the Board of Health's view that there should be an independent medical manpower planning mechanism. The system whereby individual practices recruited specialists to increase the range of services that group could offer led to duplication of skills, and a wasteful use of skilled manpower, procedures were being offered by those less capable of delivering them, and there was a failure to meet the overall health needs of the island. Most groups countered that centralised medical manpower planning was an intrusion upon their independent rights to practice.

Such differences led to inevitable tensions. As often happens in such circumstances in Guernsey, an outside expert was consulted. A major review of the clinical aspects of medical practice was undertaken by Sir Douglas Black and a team of specialists in 1984. The report, published early in 1985, expressed concern at the lack of manpower planning, and suggested the appointment of a Medical Advisory Committee to promote better communication with the Board. This committee was to contain representatives of the States doctors, those in private practice (both primary care and specialists) and nursing representatives.

Mr John Ferguson (a surgeon) was elected Chairman, and attempted to work with the Board of Health to resolve some of the contradictions inherent in the system. Although there was concern expressed, and much discussion between 1985 and 1989, there was little real change. The need for change was acknowledged, but no one seemed capable of initiating this.

The directive for change

At the States meeting in November 1989 the Board of Health under the presidency of Conseiller John Henry, presented a Billet d'Etat entitled *"Healthcare in Guernsey Future Planning and Funding"*. When introducing this Report to the States, Conseiller Henry stated.

"It is no good leaving things as they are because we already cannot meet the demands placed upon our service". He felt that the people of Guernsey would not welcome an NHS type service, with the possibility of two tier healthcare developing. He acknowledged the good aspects of the system as it existed, and stated that he would prefer to see change introduced, rather than starting afresh. One proposition was to privatise the Princess Elizabeth Hospital, but he felt that any such development would need to be accompanied by a compulsory health insurance scheme.

Conseiller Bob Chilcott, President of the States Insurance Authority at this time, initially lacked enthusiasm for the Report, which he felt *'contained a lot of history and not a lot of proposal for change'*. He was however encouraged by Conseiller Henry's introduction to the Report and in a robust reply, he gave his full support to compulsory insurance and moved that the Board of Health return to the States of Guernsey as quickly as possible with definite plans.

Privately he made it known that unless there was radical change he would challenge the Board of Health at the next States meeting. The States Insurance Authority in turn submitted a report to the States in March 1990, and gained States approval to *"direct the States Board of Health that when reporting to the States with details of its proposals for the introduction of charges for acute services to include in that report its conclusion on the feasibility of alternative methods of offering general practice and specialist care and including, if thought appropriate, the direct employment of qualified medical practitioners by the States whose services would be available to the public at such charges as the States may from time to time determine".*

The message to the medical profession was clear, - the system could not fail to address the need for change,- it was either *"change yourself or the matter will be taken from your hands".*

The plan for change

The Board of Health had limited time to suggest acceptable alternatives. Some of the problems rested within the medical profession, particularly, the problem of specialist re-organisation. Many doctors wanted the system to remain essentially the same, whilst others accepted the need for change. Amongst the specialists working in the group practices, some were fully accredited in their speciality whilst others were not. Some wished to split, others wished to preserve the status quo. By reason of their numerical supremacy, the final decision rested with the general practitioners, most of whom wished to preserve the 'specialists within group practice' structure. It seemed difficult to envisage how change could be achieved through democratic means. The directive and the implied threat from the States Insurance Authority was the catalyst that made change possible.

The Medical Advisory Committee and the Medical Staff Committee, under the Chairmanships of Mr John Ferguson and Dr Nigel Byrom respectively, both specialists, balloted the medical profession with regard to setting up a separate Specialist Group. It was perceived by some that a separation could have severe financial consequences upon certain groups of individual doctors. No consensus developed from the ballot. The interest of the specialists and the interests of the general practitioners were clearly separate.

The main drive for specialist separation rested with the surgical disciplines. These specialists could not conceive an integrated economical specialist service based upon the group practice system. They were aware of the situation in Canada where separation had occurred some years previously, and both sides had been slow to forgive their colleagues. Primary care doctors responded to the situation by forming a Primary Care Committee which covered the interests and the aspirations of the Islands general practitioners. The Medical Advisory Committee asked each speciality group, including primary care, for their views. The results could not have been more disparate. The surgeons and the gynaecologists favoured separation, the Primary Care Group for maintaining the group practices, whilst physicians and anaesthetists remained somewhat undecided.

The Board of Health offered to attach the professions response as an Appendix to its own Billet in order that the doctors views could be made known to the States and considered during the debate.

The Medical Staff Committee worked hard to attempt to integrate the professions several views contained in a letter to Conseiller Henry. In reply he wrote, *"I have to say at the outset that the Board of Health was most disappointed that the proposed Appendix to the Board's report did not contain more firm recommendations and a commitment to the setting up of a separate specialist practice within a stated time scale".*

He added *"The Board does not consider the proposed Appendix in its present form would be successful in convincing the States of Guernsey that the profession has accepted the need for change and is committed to progression of such a change in the near future. Indeed the Board considers that to publish the Appendix in its present form would be possibly damaging to the profession and to the Board of Health. We must ask you to consider very carefully how the case can he strengthened".*

Thus it was both political and professional pressures from the surgical specialists, that finally convinced the profession that change could not be avoided. After much further debate and discussion (sometimes heated and acrimonious), the professions response was summarised in a letter to Conseiller Henry dated the 25th July 1990, from Dr Nigel Byrom, then Chairman of the Medical Advisory Committee. It stated *"The profession recommends the development of an independent specialist practice by 1992. The specialist practice should include all surgeons, all gynaecologists, all physicians and all anaesthetists working in the group practices and in the hospital. The specialist group would be willing and responsible for the provision of a paediatric service".*

The Board of Health only reported back to the States' in October 1990 in respect of the feasibility of alternative methods of providing general practice and specialist care. They sought to retain the existing system within clearly defined conditions and recommended the setting up of a specialist practice separate from primary care. It was envisaged that primary care practices could achieve economies if certain mergers took place. The Board recommended a period of stability for five years to allow these changes to occur. The States of Guernsey at their October meeting duly agreed the Board of Health's proposals.

The Specialist Group

Once the States' had endorsed the Board proposals, change occurred rapidly. Specialists were reorganised into one group to serve the whole Island. The group commenced practice in January 1992, and recruited a Specialist Orthopaedic Surgeon, able to start a joint replacement service for the island. As this work rapidly expanded, a second Orthopaedic Surgeon was soon required.

The group worked initially from the old Grande Maison Road surgery, which they had been able to rent from the Board of Health under its new President Conseiller Bob Chilcott. The building was rapidly adapted and although appearing small from the exterior, seemed much larger once inside. Every inch of loft space was utilised, although this was not declared to the Board of Health for fear of attracting extra rent. These cramped working conditions encouraged a certain camaraderie which was helpful in bonding the group together. Many had come from different practices, often with their personal secretaries, and many new relationships needed to be forged.

Fortunately the group were soon able to purchase a site near the hospital and work was quickly underway towards the construction of the Medical Specialist Centre named Alexandra House after the nursing home which had stood on that site. It was coincidentally the birthplace of Conseiller Chilcott.

The Medical Specialist Centre, Alexandra House, was officially opened by the Bailiff on 10th July 1993. This building allowed the specialists to work in teams and to provide an integrated specialist service for the whole Island. New appointments were made following similar procedures to UK Consultant appointments in the NHS, with an external assessor from the relevant Royal College. The President of the Board of Health was also in attendance at the interview committee.

The new structure of the specialist teams within the medical specialist group has allowed expansion of specialist services and the group to date has continued to be able to attract well qualified specialists in spite of some shortages within the UK.

Great changes have occurred during the last quarter of the millennium. These changes have allowed primary care practitioners to now develop independently of their specialist colleagues. Through a combination of medical and political pressure there has been radical restructuring of all medical services. These changes would not have been achieved had the profession been left to itself. The political pressure enabled doctors and the Board of Health to work together to devise a system which has remained special for Guernsey.

The specialist services are a true secondary referral service, and it is hoped that the best features of traditional Guernsey practice have been retained, whilst necessary economies have been achieved so that the new structures will prove both flexible and robust enough to meet the changes and challenges of the new millennium.

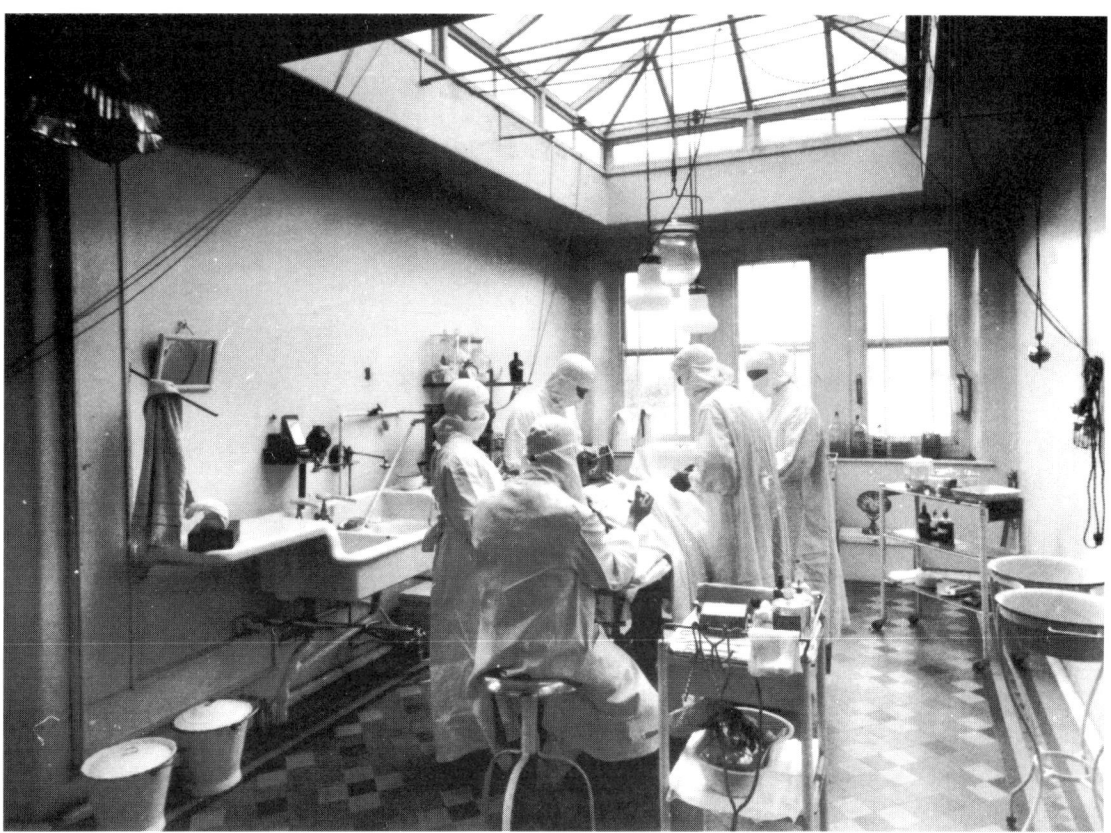

Surgery in Guernsey at the Country Hospital around 1949 and at the PEH around 1980 (Chapter Ten)

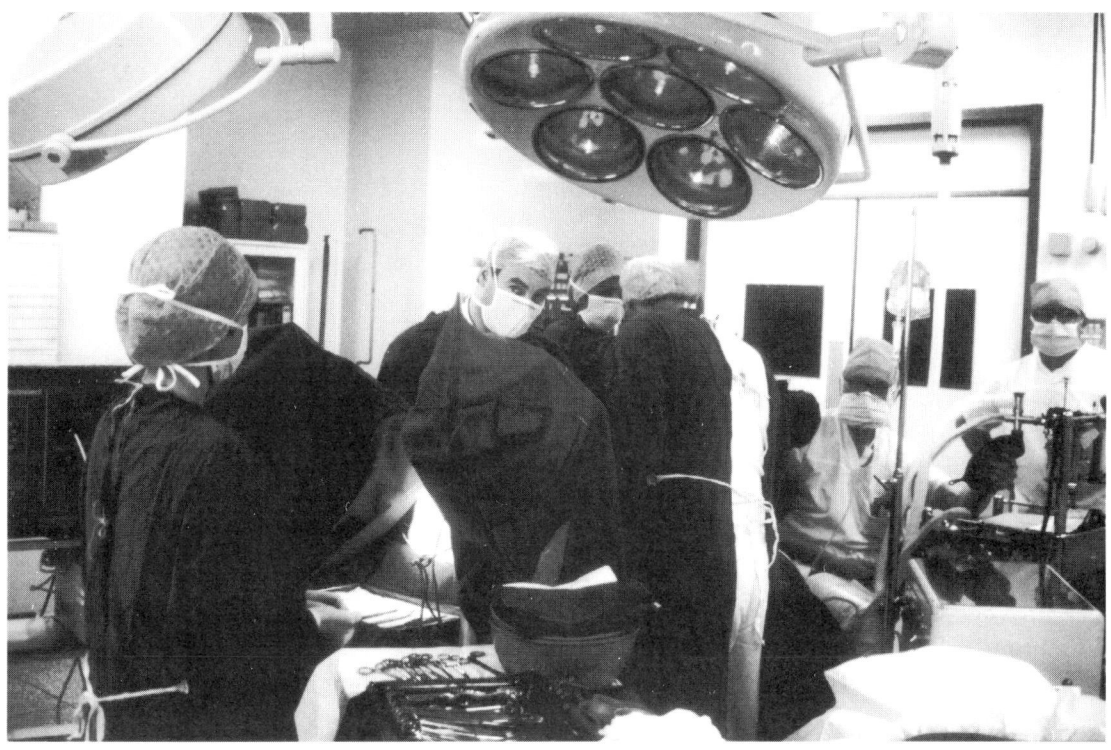

120

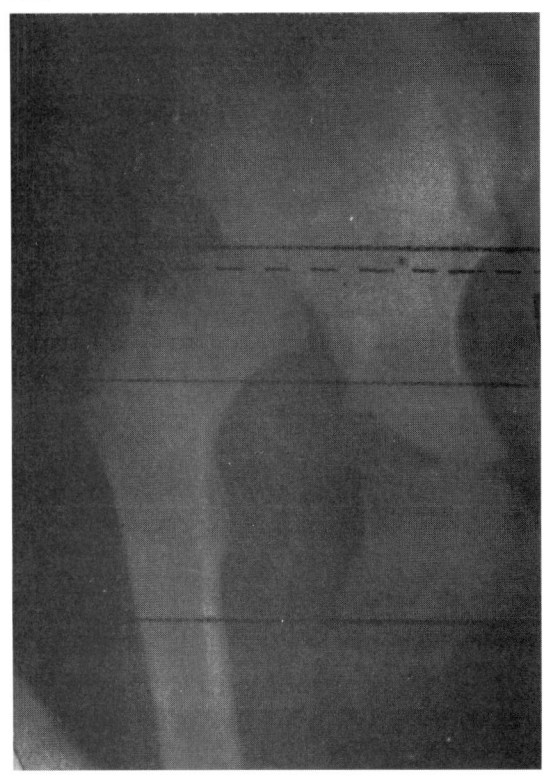

X-ray of the left hip showing a dislocation, - an original glass x-ray plate taken by Mr Rylatt for Dr C Carey around 1919 - one of the first x-rays in Guernsey. (Chapter Ten)

Bailiff Sir Graham Dorey accompanied by the late Lady Penny Dorey opening the Medical Specialist Group's new premises at Alexandra House, watched by MSG Chairman Mr Roger Allsopp. (Chapter Eleven)

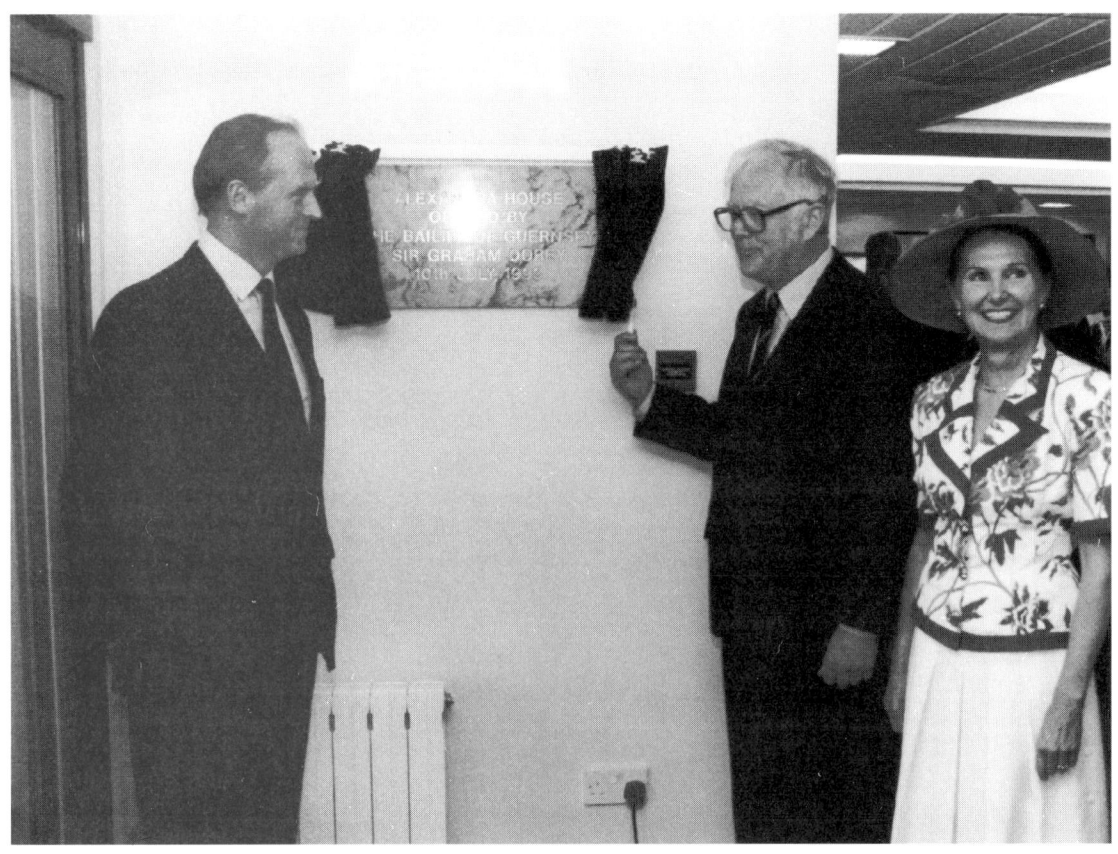

Chapter Twelve

Paying for health

S R Langford PhD

The increasing complexities of health care led inevitably to escalating costs. Following the separation of secondary care under the Medical Specialist Group the 1991 Census suggested that a sizeable minority of Guernsey's population might be excluded from seeking necessary specialist care by financial barriers. The changing philosophies of health care funding in Guernsey are explored and the pressures which led to the development and implementation of the Health Insurance Scheme explained.

Paying for health

Who should pay for health care is an emotive and frequently controversial subject wherever one lives. This was certainly the case in Guernsey in the period from the end of the Second World War until the mid-1990s when the Specialist Health Insurance Scheme was introduced. Nevertheless, there still remain anomalies in the funding of health services, notably in respect of long-term care, although it is to be hoped that these too can be resolved in the near future.

Throughout most of this century, Guernsey has had a private medical system in which the majority of doctors (including all GPs and most specialists) have remained in private practice. Nurses and many other health professionals, on the other hand, have been employed predominantly by the Board of Health (BoH), with their services being funded by the taxpayer. Consequently, charges have been raised for medical services, but not for many other health services, although BoH charging policies have varied from time to time.

The incremental development of health care provision in Guernsey has meant that the means of paying for health care have often been complex, varying depending on the service in question, and often leading to confusion for the patient. It is, therefore, interesting to note that there are now very few services for which the patient is required to pay the full economic cost; and even where this occurs then there is normally States' assistance available for those with limited financial resources. More commonly, the States, via the BoH, provides the service free at the point of delivery, funded either from taxation receipts (General Revenue) - an example being Community Nursing Services - or from a combination of General Revenue and social security contributions, e.g. specialist medical care. Alternatively, the patient pays a reduced charge for the service, the shortfall being made up from an indirect subsidy from General Revenue, e.g. BoH charges for long-term nursing care, or from a combination of General Revenue and social security contributions, e.g. the provision of drugs and medicines under the Pharmaceutical Service.

This protection of the public against the very high costs of providing health care is however, a comparatively recent development albeit with a long and complicated history. This chapter traces the development and introduction of various schemes of financial assistance which have increasingly moved the burden of paying for health care from the individual receiving the service to the community as a whole.

Post Second World War funding arrangements

At the end of the Second World War, the States provided hospital services for surgical, medical, maternity, mental health and infectious cases. With the exception of patients in the Isolation Hospital (King Edward VII Sanatorium) where there were no charges, patients were expected to pay a standard charge, or a contribution based on their declared means. The States provided radiology and pathology services, which were also charged for based on a test of the individual's means.

In addition to hospital charges, fees were payable for hospital attendances by doctors who were in private practice - and for general practice consultations, the doctors providing these services usually being one and the same. However, poor people could receive drugs, dental and ophthalmic treatment free of charge; and free medical and surgical treatment was available to poor persons through the Parish Doctor and the Island Surgeon, although the system was unpopular amongst both patients and doctors alike. Doctors did not like losing longstanding patients who could no longer afford to pay their fees and would, therefore, often not charge for their services. Patients were embarrassed by their inability to pay fees and would often make great sacrifices in order to be able to do so and thereby retain contact with the doctor of their choice.

Advent of the National Health Service

The establishment of the National Health Service in the UK, prompted the States to consider the appropriateness of a similar scheme for Guernsey, foreshadowing the development of today's Specialist Health Insurance Scheme. In November 1947, the States resolved:

> "To request the States Insurance Authority [SIA] to report to the States as soon as possible after the inauguration of the proposed Health Services Scheme in the United Kingdom as to the desirability of instituting in this Island a Health Services Scheme providing medical and hospital treatment for all persons in the community."

The SIA reported back to the States in March 1951, commenting that it was satisfied that a large number of Islanders were in a favour of a comprehensive and universal scheme of free health care based on that introduced in the UK. However, the SIA added:

> "... it is an ideal to which we subscribe, but the ideal is not always capable of being implemented, and that which is capable of implementation is not always ideal or equitable."

Having costed such a scheme, the SIA estimated that it would have to raise an additional £250,000 in taxation to fund it and concluded that, in the circumstances, it would be impractical to embark on a comprehensive scheme at that time. A limited scheme costing an additional £50,000 was, however, put forward to cover GP services, hospital and certain specialist services, midwifery services and a pharmaceutical service. This scheme was only to apply to persons (and their dependants) with an income of less than £468 per annum. They would fund the scheme by paying a weekly contribution of 10d for males and 8d for females.

This scheme was not, however, acceptable to the States, who instead resolved to request the BoH and SIA to report back jointly on a Health Services Scheme with recommendations on the services to be provided under the scheme, the persons to be covered by it, *"the desirability and practicality of requiring that some or part of the expenses be borne by the patient"*, and *"some estimate of the cost to the States"*.

The proposed 1959 Scheme

The report requested by the States in 1951 did not materialise until some eight years later, following what were described as *"long and difficult negotiations"*: the report makes interesting reading, not least because the issues raised resurfaced during the early 1990s.

The report examined a number of health care systems in other parts of the world but concluded that Guernsey should evolve *"a scheme which had no true counterpart elsewhere"*. Helpfully, it set out the principles upon which a scheme should be based namely:

> *"(i) No person should ignore actual or suspected ill-health or incapacity because he or she fears the cost of examination or treatment.*
>
> *(ii) The same standard of treatment should be available to all members of the community.*
>
> *(iii) There should be a freedom of choice on the part of the doctor and patient.*
>
> *(iv) No comprehensive scheme should be introduced which will create the impression that the facilities provided are free. On the contrary, the scheme should be so devised that the participants will realise that the cost has to be met by all persons in the community, directly and indirectly.*
>
> *(v) The difficulty of introducing a comprehensive scheme, especially a medical scheme, no matter how much it may appeal to the community and to the States, unless it meets with the approval of the Island doctors."*

The last point was the stumbling block: the two committees proposed a comprehensive scheme covering hospital services (including radiology and pathology) for which all charges were to be abolished, medical services (GP services and hospital surgery), together with a limited pharmaceutical service. This was to be funded by a mixture of social security contributions from both employers and employees, General Revenue and patient co-payments for certain services. Agreement could not, however, be reached with the doctors, primarily over the funding of the scheme.

The doctors wished to continue to receive remuneration based on the existing "fee for service" arrangements as they were concerned that their workload would significantly increase if perceived "free" medical services were provided. The two committees, on the other hand, wanted to fix the amount of money to be paid to the doctors under the scheme in order to limit the States' liability, whilst recompensing the doctors for the loss of their existing income. The two sides thus reached an impasse. (It is interesting to note that the fixed price contracts concluded with the Medical Specialist Group, Ophthalmic Group and Guernsey Physiotherapy Group addressed these issues a quarter of a century later, when it was much easier to model the effects of increased demand and its financial consequences.)

In addition, while the SIA and BoH wanted the scheme to be compulsory, the doctors argued that participation should be voluntary, (again pre-empting the debates in the 1990s as to whether Islanders should be able to opt out of the proposed schemes discussed at that time, or be required to contribute in order to ensure that the risk was shared amongst the maximum number of contributors in order to keep contributions to as low a level as possible.)

This failure to reach agreement was a great disappointment to the SIA and BoH. They considered the major funding problem to be the cost of doctors' fees, and alleged that many poor people, especially the aged, did not receive adequate medical attention as a consequence. However, without cover for these fees, the committees decided that they could not recommend the abolition of hospital charges, with the exception of those for radiology and pathology services.

The doctors, on the other hand, disputed that patients' main worry was their bills, accepting nevertheless that this was a problem from time to time. They stated that patients were also troubled by the accounts for hospital charges, particularly after prolonged bouts of illness. The doctors would, therefore, have preferred a limited scheme to cover those charges (including radiology and pathology services), plus a medical scheme for what would now be termed Supplementary Beneficiaries.

There was also a difference of opinion over the introduction of a pharmaceutical service. The SIA and BoH wanted to limit this to the supply of certain pain-killing and life-prolonging drugs, which would be provided at subsidised cost, i.e. not free. The doctors were concerned, however, that such a scheme would have no cost certainty or controls, and that it was impossible to predict which life-saving drug would be available in the future and thus covered under the scheme.

Faced with these strong and apparently irreconcilable differences of opinion, the States thus resolved:

> *"1. That the present method of assessing hospital charges be retained until it is possible to introduce the payment of weekly contributions to be used towards the cost of health services provided by the States.*
>
> *2. That all charges for X-ray and pathological examinations be abolished immediately.*

> 3. To take note of the recommendations for the introduction of a limited Pharmaceutical Service and to request that ...[the SIA and BoH] submit proposals with proper estimates of costs in regard thereto to the States ....
>
> 4. To accept in principle the introduction of a Medical Service for non-contributory pensioners and persons in similar circumstances and to request ...[the SIA and BoH] to submit proposals in regard thereto to the States.
>
> 5. To request ... [the SIA and BoH] to examine any suggestions which may lead to the creation of a Medical Service applicable to all persons ordinarily resident in Guernsey."

Abolition of Hospital Charges and the introduction of a Pharmaceutical Service

In 1966, the SIA and BoH recommenced discussions with representatives of the local division of the British Medical Association (BMA) concerning the introduction of a Health Scheme; but the only major development during the 1960s was the abolition of acute hospital charges in the public wards of the Princess Elizabeth, Castel and Maternity Hospitals with effect from 1 January 1969. The reason was that discussions had continued to be difficult; indeed, so difficult, that in January 1969 it was decided that it was not possible to reach a consensus on a comprehensive Health Scheme, and that efforts should be concentrated on developing a pharmaceutical service in view of the rapidly increasing cost and use of drugs.

Three months into these limited discussions, the doctor representatives resigned from the Working Party established for this purpose, unable to continue facing what for them was *"an increasing and unacceptable sense of frustration"*: they were unable to be replaced but the Working Party continued on regardless.

The root of the problem was the threat that a third party, i.e. the States, would interfere with a doctor's clinical freedom to prescribe through the imposition of administrative arrangements to contain and monitor expenditure on drugs and medicines. This was explained fully in the SIA's report to the States in January 1972, wherein it was reported that of the 35 practising doctors there were *"many who would reject the recommendations completely and only a few who would accept them without revision"*. Indeed, the two doctors on the BoH also dissented from the SIA proposals.

Despite the doctors' opposition, the States accepted the SIA's recommendations for the introduction of a pharmaceutical service (which came into operation in June 1973) funded by weekly social security contributions, prescription charges and a grant from General Revenue. The doctors' refusal to operate a scheme based on a "Prescribed List" of drugs was, however, taken into account, and "Open List" prescribing recommended.

This remains the basis of the Scheme in operation today, with very few drugs or medicines being excluded from general prescription. Prescription charges payable by the patient remain very low compared with the UK at £1.80 per item, particularly when one considers that expenditure on the pharmaceutical service totalled £9.55 million in 1998, income from prescription charges being £765,000. (Social Security contributions to fund this scheme are included with contributions to fund other health service benefits, as discussed overleaf.)

Cost concerns in the 1980s

The 1980s were characterised by increasing concerns about the cost of health care, predominantly rapid increases in BoH expenditure, but also, from the middle of the decade, concerns about the cost of doctors' fees.

In its 1983 report to the States on hospital fees, the BoH made it clear that it was considering reintroducing acute hospital charges for accommodation and hospital services (e.g. food and laundry), and this received strong support from the Advisory and Finance Committee:

> *"In 1983 the estimated cost of hospital and other services provided by the Board of Health is £12.4 M of which only £500,000 will be recovered in charges. This leaves a net cost to the taxpayer of £11.9 M or about £4.28 per week, for every man, woman and child of the resident population or about £8 per week for every man and woman of the 'working population'. This cost will clearly rise, both through inflation and through an increase in the number of older, retired persons in the Island. In the opinion of the Advisory and Finance Committee serious consideration must be given to increasing revenue from charges as opposed to taxes wherever this can be done without causing undue hardship or deflecting the object of the service concerned."*

In 1985, a review team led by Sir Douglas Black, made a significant, albeit passing, reference to reports of the high costs of fees for specialist medical care, and anomalies in funding arrangements, which could provide *'financial disincentives to taking up health care"*. The review team recommended the BoH to consider alternative or additional methods of funding health care in the Island.

These separate concerns were drawn together in a report from the Advisory and Finance Committee considered by the States in July 1986, which subsequently commissioned a report by Peat Marwick Mitchell (PMM) to look at:

> *"a) a coherent policy relating to charges for services;*
>
> *b) methods of paying such charges;*
>
> *c) to what extent the insurance principle may be adequate to meet the needs of the population."*

Before, however, this report was received, the SIA decided that the difficulties being experienced by some Islanders in meeting doctors' fees, especially for specialist and surgical procedures, had reached such a level that a specific scheme had to be introduced to ensure these costs did not deter people from seeking necessary treatment:

> *"Inability to pay for treatment, which if not carried out could seriously affect a person's quality of life and long-term good health, is not something that this community should tolerate in 1987."*

The SIA, therefore, proposed the introduction of an interim scheme of discretionary loans and grants - the Medical Expenses Assistance Scheme (MEAS) - to cover that section of the community not provided for under statutory schemes of assistance, (e.g. Supplementary Benefit, Public Assistance, Industrial Medical Benefit). The MEAS scheme would be available to assist with the costs of surgical and other specialist procedures, and the high costs of primary care, especially when combined with such procedures[1].

The PMM report was published later in 1987. Amongst its conclusions was the following statement:

> "1. The cost of health care (partly arising from medical expectations and partly as a result of developments in medical technology) places a considerable burden on the States and individual patients. The need to tackle this is urgent."

PMM thus examined and costed three options that could be considered by the States;

1. A compulsory States-run insurance scheme to cover either primary care or primary and secondary care costs;

2. A voluntary Island-wide insurance scheme run by a private insurer, but with financial incentives from the States to make premiums attractive to encourage a high participation rate;

3. A voluntary Island-wide insurance scheme allowing the individual to select his own insurer, but again with financial incentives from the States to encourage high take-up.

Before, however, the BoH could respond to these proposals, the SIA's proposals for the introduction of grants for GP and nurse consultations in the surgery or at home were accepted by the States. In making these proposals, the SIA acknowledged that the main issue was the cost of specialist treatment, but nevertheless saw this as a step towards implementing the PMM report.

These health benefit grants remain in place today, although their value has remained the same - £8 for a doctor consultation, £4 for a nurse consultation. At the time of their introduction the "£8 grant" represented more than half the private consultation fee; but this has now reduced to a third (standard consultation fee £25-£26).

A Health Insurance Scheme gains momentum

The PMM report had provided some impetus for the introduction of some form of health insurance scheme, but before this could seriously be considered the BoH felt it necessary to establish the basis on which services were to be delivered. Two reports on this matter were considered by the States - firstly in November 1989, and secondly in October 1990.

---

[1] The MEAS scheme remains in operation today, albeit in a reduced form following the introduction of the Specialist Health Insurance Scheme. It is now used predominantly to assist with paying for the high costs of dental treatment. Expenditure on the scheme in 1998 was £43,000.

In the first report, the BoH and the doctors allied to state their belief in the right of every patient to receive the treatment they required without fear of rationing on cost grounds.

The BoH report also gave qualified support to the insurance concept being investigated by the SIA; but made it clear that, in the BoH's view, the scheme must be compulsory, with those who could afford to pay for insurance themselves doing so. It, therefore, favoured a privately-run scheme, which included cover for hospital charges, warning that if services were free at the point of delivery demand could be unlimited.

The States accepted the principles espoused by the BoH and resolved:

> "1. That residents of Guernsey and Alderney shall continue to have access to Health Care Services without the imposition by the States of arbitrary financial or other constraints until such time as the Board of Health have determined and the States have approved charges for hospital services.
>
> 2. That the States Board of Health shall report to the States as soon as may be with details of its proposals for the introduction of charges for such services.
>
> 3. That to enable persons using such services to pay charges -
>
>   (a) all residents of Guernsey and Alderney should be required to have health insurance to meet the costs of their own medical and health care and that of their dependants;
>
>   (b) that the States shall assist those who for whatever reason are unable to obtain adequate insurance to provide for themselves and their dependants;
>
> 4A. To request the States Insurance Authority to report to the States as soon as the States have accepted the proposals of the Board of Health for the introduction of charges for acute services with details and costs of suitable health insurance schemes which would include cover for charges made for acute hospital services."

However, in early 1990, before either committee could report back to the States, the BMA announced a 12% increase in surgical fees and a 30% increase in GP consultation fees. The SIA immediately reported these developments to the States, concerned that they would erode the value of the health benefit grant before it was introduced (in 1991) and increase the contributions payable to fund an insurance scheme. The SIA thus recommended and the States agreed:

> "To direct the States Board of Health that when reporting to the States with details of its proposals for the introduction of charges for acute services to include in that report its conclusions on the feasibility of alternative methods of providing general practice and specialist cure including, if thought appropriate, the direct employment of qualified medical practitioners by the States whose services would be available to the public at such charge as the States may from time to time determine."

Subsequently, in October 1990, the States considered a further report from the BoH which compared the island's system of service delivery and funding with the UK and Jersey. The BoH concluded that *"if present concern relates solely to the doctors' charges and about how these can be met then this is the problem which needs to be solved, and that it will not be solved by totally changing the Island's health care system."*

The BoH did, however, recommend one major change to the system of health care delivery, whereby the Specialists would separate from their group practices (delivering a mixture of GP and specialist services) to form a single group of their own. The BoH stated that this would be significant from a funding point of view, because the new group would set its own fees and had given a commitment to introduce package prices for certain procedures as soon as possible. This split would, therefore, assist the SIA in bringing forward proposals for a health insurance scheme.

The States agreed to this change in arrangements and awaited reports from the SIA and BoH on the introduction of hospital charges and an insurance scheme to fund these and other doctors' fees.

Health Insurance Scheme proposals

These proposals came forward in April 1992. The SIA recommended adoption of a comprehensive scheme to cover acute primary and secondary medical care costs, plus hospital charges to be introduced by the BoH for inpatient services, day patient attendances, outpatient treatments, theatres, radiology and pathology services, pre- and post-natal maternity care and surgical implants. The scheme would also cover, amongst other things, certain treatments in UK hospitals, terminal care costs, accommodation charges in private nursing homes, some limited physiotherapy and osteopathy treatments, medical referrals for chiropody and dietetics, oral surgical operations for impacted wisdom teeth, repatriation costs, rehabilitation costs and essential ambulance journeys. Co-payments were to be required from patients for primary care, osteopathy and physiotherapy consultations (£5), home visits (£10), and nurse consultations (£3).

The proposed scheme *"to relieve people of the burden of meeting medical and other bills at the time of illness"* was to be compulsory and would cover all islanders after 26 weeks residence, with no exclusions for pre-existing medical conditions.

The scheme was to be administered by the SIA, but following a competitive tendering exercise, the insurer was to be Norwich Union Healthcare Limited, initially under a 4 year contract. The total cost of the contract was estimated as £28.01 million, of which £14.2 million was to cover hospital charges. Social security contributions would, therefore, have to rise by 2.3%, split equally between employer and employee, in order to fund the scheme; there would also be a need for a grant from General Revenue of £18.71 million. The maximum additional contribution was thus to be £9.04 per week for a self-employed person, £4.52 per week for an employer or employee. Contributions were also to be required from persons over the age of 65 on an income-related basis.

The proposals prompted a lengthy States' debate and, although it was agreed that the BoH could introduce hospital charges once a health insurance scheme was in place, the States did not agree to the SIA concluding and reporting back on the final details of its contract negotiations with Norwich Union. Instead, the States resolved;

> "1. To agree in principle that there should be established a Health Insurance Scheme; and
>
> 2. To direct the States Insurance Authority to report back to the States ... with recommendations for a Health Insurance Scheme taking full account of the various issues raised during the debate..."

The major concerns referred to included the compulsory element - many Islanders already having private health insurance that they wished to retain; the relinquishing of administrative responsibility to an external body; the overall costs of the scheme, in particular the transfer of hospital costs and the charges to be introduced therefor from General Revenue to insurance contributions; the perceived low premiums in the first year; and thus the problems of containing costs and premiums in the face of escalating demand once services were perceived as free (albeit that patients would receive copies of all "bills", and managed care and best practice protocols would be put in place).

Having taken account of these concerns and consulted widely, the Guernsey Social Security Authority (GSSA) (formerly SIA) reported back to the States in January 1994, reaffirming its conviction that an Island-wide insurance scheme offered the *"best opportunity to protect the population against medical bills which they cannot afford while at the same time allowing closer control on health care spending."* The GSSA put forward three options for consideration:

1. A scheme covering hospital services, primary and specialist medical care;

2. A scheme covering primary and specialist medical care;

3. A scheme covering specialist medical care only.

The GSSA recommended the third option, known as "Option A": partly because the BMA opposed the inclusion of primary care in the scheme, believing the major concerns to relate to the high costs of specialist care bills; partly because private insurers supported the "freedom of choice lobby" and a specialist only scheme would leave business for the private insurers; and partly because the BoH believed that there was no longer any requirement to introduce hospital charges to control expenditure on acute hospital services.

The revised scheme was thus much smaller in scope and significantly far less costly than the Norwich Union scheme. The estimated costs of all health benefits in 1995 was £15.35 million, of which the Specialist Health Insurance Scheme cost was £5.0 million. Contributions to fund the scheme were limited to a 1% increase, giving an estimated maximum weekly contribution of £4.14 per week for a self-employed person, £2.07 per week each for an employer and his employee. These costs were to be contained by entering into fixed price, fixed term, contracts with specialist providers, notably the Medical Specialist Group (MSG) which had come into existence in 1992.

This more limited scheme found virtually unanimous favour with the States, which approved Option A in principle, instructing the GSSA to report back with final details of the scheme based on that option. The proposal to re-introduce hospital charges was thus abandoned; although the States did accept an amendment that left open the possibility of the scheme being extended to cover primary care fees, by requiring the GSSA to report on the feasibility of this option once the specialist scheme had been in force for a period of 12 months. In 1995, this Resolution was rescinded, although the GSSA is not debarred from reporting back to the States on this matter should circumstances change at any point in the future[2].

The Specialist Health Insurance Scheme

There then followed 17 months of intensive and complicated negotiations between the GSSA, the BoH and the MSG over the terms of the contract that would form the main basis of the Specialist Health Insurance Scheme that came into operation on 1 January 1996.

These negotiations are described in some detail in the GSSA's report to the States in June 1995 that set out the heads of agreement in that contract. The proposed scheme was to be based on a 7 year contract between the States and the MSG, the annual costs for which were fixed at £4.73 million (in 1994 values), with annual variations to take account of movements in the Guernsey Retail Price Index. Broadly speaking, the contract was to provide insurance cover for all residents of Guernsey and Alderney for all consultations and surgical procedures undertaken at the Group's clinic and in hospitals managed by the BoH in Guernsey and Alderney. In addition, as part of the contract, the MSG agreed to accept various quality standards regarding matters such as maximum waiting times for consultations and inpatient treatment.

The scheme was to be funded through increased social security contributions, payable by employers, employees, self-employed and non-employed persons: the former three categories on an earnings-related basis, the latter on an income-related basis. Significantly, two new groups of contributors were created; namely, persons aged 65 and over and non-married women not in employment, each with a personal income above an annual income threshold of £6,500. Contributions would rise by 1%, shared equally between employers and employees, at a maximum weekly contribution of £2.13 per week (£4.26 in aggregate).

This scheme was acceptable to the States, who consented to an agreement being concluded with the MSG on the terms set out in the GSSA's report. In addition, the States consented to the GSSA and BoH negotiating and agreeing contracts for ophthalmic services and physiotherapy associated with specialist care.

A contract with the Ophthalmic Group covering consultations and treatment at their clinic and in hospital was speedily concluded in time for the launch of the scheme on 1 January 1996, but negotiations with the Physiotherapists proved more difficult and were not finally concluded until 1997. (Indeed, in March 1997, negotiations having broken down, it was proposed that the BoH employ or contract its own physiotherapists to deliver inpatient and post- discharge physiotherapy services under the Specialist Health Insurance Scheme. This, however, was rejected by the States and negotiations recommenced.)

---

[2] GPs remain in private practice and charge on a fee per item of service basis. The current fee for a surgery consultation is £25.26; a home visit starts at £50.52. GPs also charge for providing cover for the Accident and Emergency Department at the Princess Elizabeth Hospital.

The contract with the Guernsey Physiotherapy Group covers specialist inpatient physiotherapy in hospital and post-discharge physiotherapy when this is necessary as part of a specialist medical procedure[3].

Effects of the Specialist Health Insurance Scheme

The Specialist Health Insurance Scheme introduced a new range of health benefits - specialist medical, ophthalmic and physiotherapy - for all residents of the island. In 1998, the value of these benefits was £6.07 million.

The maximum contribution to fund this scheme and other health benefits - the health benefit grants and the pharmaceutical service - is currently £12.56 per week, of which £4.83 per week funds the Specialist Health Insurance Scheme benefits. For this weekly contribution, residents receive the services covered by the various contracts free at the point of delivery. There has been no increase in the percentage contribution rate required since the Scheme's inception in 1996.

Long-term Care Services

The focus of this article has been payments for acute medical care: space has not permitted discussion of the payment/funding arrangements for services such as dentistry, osteopathy, chiropractic or community health services. Similarly, it has not been possible to trace the development of services available to Islanders through the Reciprocal Health Agreement or contractual arrangements with UK Trusts.

Of particular interest is the history of the arrangements for the funding of long-term care services (including long-term nursing care in the King Edward VII and Castel Hospitals, private residential and nursing homes, and BoH community homes for the mentally ill and persons with a learning disability). This makes an equally interesting story; and one that currently does not have such a positive ending. Readers with an interest in this subject are, therefore, referred to the Consultation Document issued by the GSSA in November 1998 entitled *"The Funding of Long-term Care and Associated Services"*.

At the time of writing, the GSSA is seeking the States' agreement in principle to proposals to introduce a long-term care insurance scheme to assist with payment of the very high charges that are made for these services. [If adopted, this will build up on the insurance principles established by the introduction of the Specialist Health Insurance Scheme.]

---

[3] While the Specialist Health Insurance Scheme covers inpatient and some post-discharge physiotherapy services, outpatient physiotherapy treatment is generally charged for on a private fee for service basis. The cost of a standard physiotherapy consultation is currently between £17 and £30.

Conclusions

The States' commitment to a health scheme of some form originated in 1947 and came to fruition in 1996. Nevertheless, just three years after the introduction of the Specialist Health Insurance Scheme, it is easy to forget the difficulties which many Islanders had faced in paying for medical care, especially specialist's bills.

The 1991 Census had shown that only 60% of the population had health insurance for specialist care. Many of those policies were characterised by exclusions or high premiums for pre-existing medical conditions, or financial limits based on the premiums selected. Expenditure on MEAS had increased 102% in real terms between 1988 and 1994; and bills of £9,000 for the care of a premature baby or over £1,000 for operations like hip replacements or hysterectomies were then commonplace. Bills of this size were, therefore, believed to act as a barrier to seeking required medical treatment, seemingly borne out by the 20% surge in demand for specialist medical services once the Specialist Health Insurance Scheme was introduced.

For many islanders, the Specialist Health Insurance Scheme has therefore been a great success, offering reassurance that the high costs of specialist medical care will be met regardless of an individual's medical problems or financial situation. Fixed term, fixed price, contracts have also provided a means of containing the costs of specialist medical services.

The next landmark in this saga will, therefore, be the renegotiation of the various contracts that make up the scheme in 2002. However, before then, it is to be hoped that the one remaining major health care funding issue - that of long-term care - will have been finally resolved to the community's satisfaction. If that can occur before the end of this millennium, Guernsey will truly have made great strides in dealing with the financial issues involved in ensuring the health and well-being of its population.

Main sources

SIA "Social Insurance" Billet d'Etat XXIX (26 November 1947), pp 519-543.

SIA "Health Services Scheme" Billet d'Etat V (7 March 1951), pp 103-105.

SIA and BoH "Health Services Scheme" Billet d'Etat IX (16 September 1959), pp 193-209.

BoH "Abolition of Hospital Charges" Billet d'Etat XVII (27 November 1968), pp 490-491.

SIA and BoH "Establishment of a Pharmaceutical Service" Billet d'Etat I (26 January 1972), pp 3-41.

BoH "Hospital Fees" Billet d'Etat XXI (30 November 1983), pp 1101-1108.

BoH "Review of the Arrangements for Health Care in Guernsey" Billet d'Etat XIII (29 May 1985), (Appendix II) after p 612.

BoH "Review of the Arrangements for Health Care in Guernsey" Billet d'Etat XIX (11

AFC "Health Care and Social Benefits - Costs and Charges" Billet d'Etat XVI (30 July 1986), pp 801-806.

AFC "Public Expenditure Review - Health Services - Interim Report" Billet d'Etat VII (25 March 1987), pp 314-319.

SIA "Payment of Medical Fees" Billet d'Etat XI (27 May 1987), pp 597-601.

SIA "Financial Assistance with Cost of Health Care" Billet d'Etat XXVII (14 December 1988), pp 1190-1203.

BoH "Health Care in Guernsey - Future Plans and Funding" Billet d'Etat XXIV (29 November 1989), pp 1203-1251.

SIA "Medical and Pharmaceutical Benefits" Billet d'Etat II (31 January 1990), pp 12-32.

SIA "Doctors' Fees" Billet d'Etat IV (28 February 1990), pp 141-142.

BoH "Health Care in Guernsey - Medical Services" Billet d'Etat XIX (31 October 1990), pp 923-983.

BoH "Health Care in Guernsey - Future Plans and Funding" Billet d'Etat VI (29 April 1992), pp 255-267.

SIA "Comprehensive Health Insurance Scheme" Billet d'Etat VI (29 April 1992), pp 268-300.

GSSA "Report on Health Insurance" Billet d'Etat II (26 January 1994), pp 7-148.

GSSA "Specialist Health Insurance Scheme" Billet d'Etat XIII (28 June 1995), pp 541-656.

GSSA "Specialist Health Insurance Scheme - Contract for Acute Hospital Physiotherapy" Billet d'Etat V (26 March 1997), pp 400-429.

GSSA "Specialist Health Insurance Scheme - Contract for Acute Hospital and Post Discharge Physiotherapy" Billet d'Etat XXII (26 November 1997), pp 1686-1699.

GSSA The Funding of Long-term Care and Associated Services - Volumes I and II (1998).

GSSA "Long-Term Care Insurance Scheme for Guernsey and Alderney" Billet d'Etat XIX (24 November 1999), pp 1284-1320.

Chapter Thirteen

'Two complementary Guernsey physicians'

Rev L G H Craske

The facts covering the evolution of health care in Guernsey over the past one hundred years are more easily recounted than depicting the human element which made such changes possible. Here two complementary portraits of two 'complementary Guernsey physicians' are included to illustrate this human dimension.

Dr Henry Draper Bishop

In 1787 when William Gardner surveyed Guernsey for the Master-General of the Ordnance, there was in the island a small and scattered population of generally ancient stock living in a thousand granite houses and cottages. The 19th century ended with an estimated population of some forty thousand. The true figure was unknown since there were large numbers of *"undesirable aliens"* and upon them no check was possible. Contributing to the known increase were English, Irish and French labourers. These quarried for granite or worked in the fields for an enlarged agricultural industry or were employed in the two ports now accustomed to increased cargoes. They were joined by compatriot butchers, bakers, grocers and other traders, who had followed to supply their needs. In addition there was an Army garrison of increased strength and a coterie with modest capital and pension which, after service on the boundaries of the Empire, had found a temperate climate, an enhanced social prominence and domestic pleasantries at less cost than in Britain. Nevertheless no one could be isolated from the stinks, pollution and disease which the growth of the population had brought.

The greatest numbers of Guernsey's thousands were crowded into the smallest, sublet houses in conditions altogether detrimental to health and where premature death was common. Tuberculosis, intimately connected with nutritional standards and ill ventilated and overcrowded housing, was virulent and a great killer. There were some decent public pumps in the town, but generally the community remained dependent upon water drawn from ancient wells and streams closely situated near pits for the disposal of excrement. Enteric fever spread by micro-organisms in water and food was exuberant, typhoid, spread by the ingesting of contaminated drink and food along with its handmaiden typhus, a rickettsial disease spread mainly by the faeces of the body louse, lurked in alleys and in ships from foreign parts, whilst dreaded and fatal among the children were scarlet fever and diphtheria, both encouraged by insanitary milk supplies.

To war against these there came in 1903 young Henry Draper Bishop. He had trained in London and Brussels writing a paper on *"Ruptured popliteal aneurysm-gangrene- late amputation and recovery"* the preparation of which was perhaps of more use to him as an Honorary Surgeon to the Guernsey Artillery?

He was to hold the post of Medical Officer of Health for many years simultaneously with his private practice at Albion Terrace, St Sampson's. The arrangement was not to the liking of his medical colleagues, but it was something both he and they had to accept owing to the unwillingness of the States of Guernsey to pay for a full-time Medical Officer.

Among them were some who were afraid that his appointment would lead to a preference in the population for his own practice and a consequent lessening in their income. This was exacerbated by a rarity in those days of Bishop's wife, Mary Frances, being herself a medical practitioner (a partnership apparently of but short duration; no mention is made of her after 1909, when it is presumed that she died, causing Bishop to move from their home Santa Monica, Vale Road, to a house in the Grange. Their only child, a daughter, married Major W Collings, son of Dr C d'A Collings.)

That the two were perceived as a threat by some of their medical colleagues is clear from a disjointed letter written by Dr Norinan Wetaker refusing an invitation to the opening of the King Edward Sanatorium in December 1902, an institution to which Bishop was to devote himself, visiting it every day for years.

Wetaker had the curious notion that *"Island medical law 'was' violated" by Bishop's part-time appointment." "Personally" he wrote "I have nothing against that gentleman but I distinctly decline to introduce Dr and Mrs Dr Bishop to any of my patients giving them an undue and unfair advantage (over) the general practitioners of this small island under the circumstances it will be impossible for any unison."*

Other examples of professional unpleasantness continued to appear, usually owing to a supposed trespassing over the boundary between private attendance on a patient and the responsibility of the Medical Officer of Health once the patient was placed in an isolation ward. In October 1905 Dr Wm. Duncan of King's Mills went to the extremity of accusing Bishop of 'stealing a patient'. This was a boy named Duquemin who was suffering from diphtheria whom Bishop had cared for in the hospital and injected with anti diphtheritic serum

"Seeing you stole my patient knowing that I was in attendance on him I look to you for payment of the fees. I was in attendance on him before he was sent to the Sanatorium. I arranged with his parents that I would attend him there: if you do not wish your conduct to be exposed you will pay it without another word." It transpired that although Duncan had told the parents that he would attend the boy, they had other ideas when the Matron told them that Bishop would do it for nothing.

Dr Charles Jones of Newington Place, an excellent, hard-working doctor among the poor of St Sampson's, more properly directed his reproaches to the Board of Health rather than to his friend Bishop. He ordered a special diet and a pint of Champagne for a poor patient seriously ill with diphtheria in the Town Isolation Hospital and found that he was required to pay for them. Anyone entering the Town Isolation Hospital at that time would have indeed needed a pint of Champagne whether he was ill or not! The place was wildly insanitary. Jones himself complains that the escape of sewer gas into the building is *"both dangerous and disgusting"*.

The duality of part-time MoH and General Practitioner continued until 1927. In that year the Board of Health sought to advertise the full-time post in *"The Lancet"*. The island's medical profession thought the salary offered was inadequate, and at its request the journal refused the advertisement.

When agreement had finally been reached, Henry Bishop was appointed and remained until his retirement in August 1935: but part-time or full-time his commitment to the reform of the public health of Guernsey was absolute and wholly admirable.

He began his work by describing himself as *"an enthusiast"* and a *"dreamer"*. An *"enthusiast"* for that Victorian sanitary movement which had come to see the connection between dirt and disease and personal hygiene and health, a *"dreamer"* of a future time when honest and hardworking patients would be free of *"rack landlords"* extorting unreasonable rents; when families would be provided with proper housing with *"satisfactory sanitary fittings"* and with *"baths and wash-houses with drying grounds"*. The enthusiasm was to roam wide. It caused a constant seeking out of polluted wells and leaking cesspits, a pleading for a better excrement disposal and a cleaner milk distribution, and a determination to reform the wholly unsatisfactory nursing institutions. He was disturbed by the number of infant deaths described as *"convulsions"* and suspected that some might have been poisonings encouraged by the custom of insuring children's lives at birth. Such infanticide and fraudulence was common in London and other cities.

Aware of it, Bishop sought reform in the Registration procedure in Guernsey where it was left to the father to report the cause of death at the Greffe. Curious happenings were also occurring in the registration of illegitimate births. In 1906 the Greffier reported only 23 in the island or a rate of 2%, when in the first seven months of that year one doctor alone in a small practice in Les Gravees had seen 24 unmarried pregnant women. His enthusiasm found its way even to the Churchyards where he found the reluctance to cover with soil previously buried coffins in poorly constructed vaults most disgusting. He complained to the Board of Health on behalf of the Rectors that they should not be subjected to such very objectionable and dangerous odours and repulsive sights.

In the early years of this century Guernsey schools were often insanitary places with contaminated well water. The cheap milk the children drank was subject to adulteration; it was the common practice of milkmen in St Peter Port to carry open barrels amongst the uncovered milk churns into which pig wash and old vegetables were thrown.

Vauvert Infant School was a startling example of insanitation. The teaching was done in two wooden enclosures, each with fifty children, with one enclosure opening directly into the two common closets. The smell was dreadful. In this enclosure there was in 1903 a serious outbreak of diphtheria, beginning among a group of children seated closest to the closets.

Three years later there was a very serious and protracted epidemic of the same disease in St Martin's School, a Parish where the general sanitary conditions were deplorable and where the Constables had ignored Bishop's demands that the polluted school well should be closed. Seventy children were taken by their teachers to file pass the corpse of one of the girls, some bending to kiss it. This thought Bishop, added another seventeen cases of diphtheria within the next fortnight.

He was adamant that the house in the Castel parish described as the "Isolation Hospital" should be replaced. Its mortuary was a storage room for blankets and its laundry both a coal store and a bathing place for fever patients. Patients complained to the Constables that their sick children sent to the Isolation Hospital by compulsory notice were returned home *"disgustingly dirty"*, *"the head in a lively condition"* and their clothing *'filthy and only fit to be burnt"*.

There were also the Island's two work-houses, each with an infirmary and an asylum attached. Bishop sought one new building with reformed care and nursing. The Castel buildings, the responsibility of the Country Parish Constables, he describes as *"in a terribly unsanitary condition unfit for human habitation and a disgrace to any civilised community"*. Inside the infirmary the patients slept on mattresses stuffed with dry seaweed, repositories of lice and microbes. There were no closets, sinks or fixed baths: the stench was awful since all motions passed during the night had to remain in the wards until morning.

On the day he arrived to make his first thorough inspection, the sixteen outdoor trough closets, filthy and smelling abominably, had been closed for two weeks. During the closure the men patients had been relieving themselves in a corner of a field, while the women were using buckets in the crowded and ill-ventilated wards. Patients complained of constant abdominal pains, vomiting and diarrhoea. He was himself violently sick during his visit and remained unwell for some days.

The disgusting odours of the Castel Hospital were to continue for some years. P.T.Mignot, the Rector of the Castel, was complaining in 1905 that its smell was so bad that he and his family were *"scarcely able to stay in the Rectory"*.

The same year that Bishop made his stringent criticism of the Castel Isolation Hospital was one of continual cold and damp which confined people to their overcrowded houses and increased the sickness and deaths from tuberculosis alarmingly. There was no known cure for this disease and all that Bishop was able to do was to issue a leaflet entitled *"Useful Hints to Consumptive Patients"*.

At the same time he risked unpopularity by mentioning to those whose indifference, culpability or ignorance persuaded them not to hear it, that while the high mortality was associated with social deprivation, ultimately tuberculosis was no respecter of class.

Such was the social dread of this disease that in later years he was hindered by the foolishness of the Guernsey Royal Court which, as in a game of *"follow my leader"*, insisted upon following the recent English law limiting the notification of the disease to *"patients of the pauper class"*.

The Medical Officer was faced with the illogicality of a law which required that rooms occupied by pulmonary consumptive sufferers should be disinfected after death, whilst provided that the sufferers were not paupers, he must remain ignorant of the whereabouts of the disease during life.

There was no public veterinary supervision in Guernsey at the turn of the century. In its absence, Bishop was moved to challenge the brutal and filthy practices in the animal slaughter houses. From these there issued daily a disgusting and unsanitary concoction of entrails and viscera mixed with blood and dung. This was loaded into horse drawn carts and driven through the streets of St Sampson's and St Peter Port to spread as manure upon the fields, the delicacy of the Town Constables prompting them to ask that these journeys should be in the evening with the contents covered.

He found that a knackery at St Sampson's situated among dwelling houses, slaughtered some three hundred horses a year together with two hundred other beasts. The effluent flowed into an open douet and then into two cesspits which were also used as latrines by the labourers The stench was horrible and overpowering. Nearby the cesspit was the skull and part of an uncleaned backbone of a horse emitting an extremely offensive odour, while spread out to dry on top of a fowl house was a large quantity of sinews and tails of animals. There was a well close by used for drinking water. He insisted that the knackery be closed as soon as the order could be made but *"soon"* was unconscionably long.

Nevertheless his strictures had brought about a wonderful improvement by 1908, when Meat Inspectors, whose vigilance he described as *"very thorough"*, were being employed to guard against the spread of tuberculosis and other diseases through the use of tainted knives to cut cattle glands and tissue. There was alarm in the previous year when bovine tuberculosis was found in two herds in the island after an exhibition of Guernsey cattle in England where they had been kept in closed buildings.

Bishop thought that the common opinion that cattle became infected whilst grazing in the fields was fallacious and that dark, ill-ventilated and foul stables ,with floors covered with filth and walls and roof space with cobwebs and dust, promoted conditions for a veritable forcing house for Tuberculosis.

In one such stable in Guernsey he placed a thermometer during a cold January night and found that the temperature rose to 72°F. The cowmen told him that in the morning they could hardly enter the sheds without vomiting. This caused him to campaign for clean, well ventilated sheds and to encourage farmers in the use of thermometers to ensure that the temperature should not exceed 50°F.

Henry Bishop died aged 70 on August 19th 1935, three weeks after his retirement. A grateful States Office presented to him, when sick in bed and confused, a Barograph to pursue his intended hobby of measuring the variations in the atmospheric pressures of the island. The Board of Health engaged a special nurse from England to nurse him during the three weeks of his illness, charging only out of pocket expenses; a small consideration now perhaps, but of significance at that time. From the beginning he was grateful for the kindness of the Board and the way in which it entered into his difficulties and stimulated him to carry out his work.

His thirty years of sanitary, hospital and social reform were not fought against the Board's obstinacy but against feudal facilities and ancient parochial arrangement that had suddenly been overtaken by demographic change. This change brought the host of acute infections common in burgeoning Victorian cities. He was to be the harbinger of the tremendous successes in controlling them; yet early he discerned that new social habits such as smoking were to bring those most frequent diseases of our own times-heart disease and cancer.

Dr Harry Bound

To deal with these and other related diseases (two million people in the United Kingdom now suffer from asthma and more than one in ten have eczema), a technology has arisen which involves an astronomical and ever-increasing expenditure. Together with the requirement for an inexhaustible treasury, there has grown a considerable unease with the absolute trust in scientific medicine leading to a call for civilised discussion with complementary therapies and other systems. The call became louder and more persistent after 1983, when the Prince of Wales was elected President of the BMA. He used the opportunity to exhort its members to re-examine the basic assumptions of technical medicine and to be more open-minded about alternatives.

The BMA had no choice but to inquire into complementary medicine. After three years it produced a report which was very defensive of scientific medicine and dismissive of alternative methods. Some of these it charged with being primitive, untested, ineffective and *"inconsistent with natural laws"*.

Its conclusions were, in turn, rudely dismissed as *"the last gasp of the dinosaurs"* and generally criticised as *"outdated"* and *"absurd"*. Complementary therapy had found much popular support during the three years taken to produce the report.

The importance of complementary methods however, had already been foreseen by a Guernsey doctor several years before the Prince of Wales made his speech. Harry Bound was Senior Partner of the La Plaiderie and Le Longfrie Practice. He joined this partnership of A.D and E.A.Bisson and J. Strickland in 1955 after work in Nigeria as a medical officer for the Colonial Medical Service.

His early days in the island were spent chiefly among the country people in the Parish of St Peter: these would have been days of that all-embracing nature then required of an island G.P., from being anaesthetist at the hospital during the day to writing and sticking stamps on monthly accounts in the evenings

Harry Bound was a devout Roman Catholic. As his spiritual interests grew so did his open questioning of obsessive medical technology with its frequent lack of heart and lack of understanding. It took courage for one who had been Chairman of the Guernsey BMA and was a Fellow of the Royal College of General Practitioners to be at the same time an inspiration for the founding of the Guernsey Association of Complementary Therapists. The medical profession for much of this century had a standing regulation that prevented a doctor from studying complementary methods which generally it shunned as quackery. In 1983 his belief that sickness had its spiritual lessons led him to join with others in founding the Guernsey Healing

Harry Bound, like Henry Bishop before him, had been a student at the Royal London Hospital. His time there was preceded by undergraduate days at Clare College, Cambridge, where he met the Reverend C.F.D Moule, Dean of the College and later Lady Margaret Professor of Divinity at the University. It was C.F.D. Moule who gave the address at the Requiem Mass at Notre Dame du Rosaire in 1997 in which he described Harry Bound's attitude to medicine as *"pastoral"* and with *"a deep concern which developed in him for what (perhaps ineptly) is often called Spiritual Healing"*. It was described by Bound himself as *"Holistic Care"*.

I am inclined myself to think of "Holistic" as a modern misnomer. Greek and Hebrew words translated by "holy" do not have anything to do with "wholeness" or "health". The idea that they did was demolished in 1961 by James Barr, Professor of Old Testament studies at the University of Edinburgh in *"The Semantics of Biblical Language"*. It is impossible to suppose that the rear chamber of the Temple in Jerusalem usually called *"the Holy of Holies"* was in fact a place specially healthy or specially 'whole', or that valuables captured by the Hebrews and devoted to the divine possession were *"healthy to the Lord"*. Nevertheless whatever we might call it, the method for which Harry Bound had a deep concern was the co-operative relationship between both conventional and complementary treatments which would lead to a harmony of body, mind, emotions and spirit. The approach of such a practitioner had been well put in 1981 in *"Health for the whole person"* by A.C. Hastings (ed).

"He is as interested in the colouring of the mood that preceded an attack of chest pain and the meaning it had for the patient as in the electrocardiographic change that followed it".

"His therapeutic approach may include a meditative technique, dietary changes and exercises to improve cardiovascular functioning; psychotherapy to mitigate the depression and rage that predispose an individual to heart attack; or pastoral counselling to help someone confront the despair that can he as lethal as anatomic pathology".

C.F.D.Moule said in his Requiem address *"there is no medical person of my acquaintance who has seemed to care more patiently and perceptively for the whole person, not only seeking to treat the symptoms, but working for peace of mind and well being in the person as a whole. I forget what exactly his own formula was; but what it amounted to, anyway, was: Aim for health, even when no cure is possible"*.

In 1995 Harry Bound was found to be suffering from cancer of the bone marrow and was required to live out what he had taught. This he did in exemplary way, and in complementary manner, resorting to the latest techniques in pain-control and giving precise details on the way his body responded to them, while at the same time using the ministry of the Church through the laying on of hands.

He wrote an account of his own last struggle after the manner of C.S. Lewis's *"Screwtape Letters"*, in which he has the Intelligence Department of the International Rebel Myeloma Army observing that with advancing years he has come to think of himself increasingly as a nice gentle, comfortable guy paying lip service to Jungian views during much of his life; oblivious that in its theatre of war, the Myeloma Army advance slowly with a preference to attack older men and farm workers, but from time to time attacking anyone.

The Commander-in-Chief of the Army, General B. Badforyou complains of the setbacks caused by *"medics of optimistic attitude, employing chemotherapy who have united with loving relationship, faith and prayer"* and declares that he likes best the ones who deny its existence, become melancholic, lose faith, or are weakened by fear.

Toward his own resistance Harry calls upon the Guardian Angels Association and its Spiritual Director, Goodasgold. In his rear-guard action he falls back on his earlier medical understanding of moving toward a harmony of body, mind, emotions and spirit, an understanding which undoubtedly was helped by the harmony of his family music group (he and his wife Pauline had eight children),and that of student days in the University Orchestra. The dedication on March 6th 1999 of the new major conference room at Les Cotils Christian Centre in St Peter Port was a suitable tribute to his memory, to his work and to his personality.

What Harry believed was not altogether something newly understood by complementary medicine. No one who is observant of life, as he was, can fail to see that in many ways, some universal and some particular, the limitations of the body, and even sickness, have an educative value. The failure of the body is not pure loss: it may have beneficial spiritual potentialities. From it there may be learnt lessons which it would be difficult to conceive being taught in other ways.

Four years before his death The British Medical Association had caught up with the new thinking, and in a new report had set out information for the medical profession recommending statutory registration of the main therapies in complementary medicine.

I have described both these two Guernsey physicians as "complementary", for had not Henry Bishop touched upon "the wholeness" of being in 1903 when he saw the relationship between better housing and the removal of the daily anxiety for the poor, between peace of mind and the ending of exorbitant rents; between "well-being", and children not being taught in crowded, stinking classrooms drinking polluted water and milk?

In Bishop's day the sweet alternative vapours of aromatherapy oils were as yet hardly known, but he did at least begin with the disinfectant, drawing the line at Carbolic Acid which he smelt one day on entering the Post Office in St Peter Port and promptly ended its use thereafter.

Chapter Fourteen

The Ambulance and Rescue Service

Neil R Tucker

That Guernsey never developed an ambulance service run by the States was largely due to the vision and drive of one islander - Reginald Blanchford - who founded a unique ambulance and rescue service covering land, sea and air. Under his successors this has developed into a comprehensive modern service which must be the envy of many other island communities around the world.

'A horse drawn cart ....'

In the year 1899, Guernsey stood on the edge of the twentieth century without an emergency ambulance service as we know it.

A horse drawn cart was used by the Town Hospital, to collect patients who could not get to the infirmary unaided, but this carried no medical equipment and no trained staff. The telephone directory gave no emergency number for the crank-handled telephones of the day to call.

A century later, at the dawn of the new millennium, one call to a dedicated ambulance control room would despatch a vehicle full of equipment, with staff able to perform techniques not even practised by nurses in hospital.

During those hundred years, the concept of an ambulance service evolved from simply a means of transporting people to a medical facility, into what could be considered a branch of the medical facility itself. And Guernsey developed a service unique to the Island.

The principle of an island-wide ambulance service was established in 1908 by the Royal Court, which supplied a new horse ambulance to the Town Hospital, *"to alleviate suffering in the transport of victims of accidents occurring in any part of the island."* This was to be free of charge, although the Poor Law Board were given discretion to charge *"the military or private people who could afford to pay"*.

A second horse and cart was run by the King Edward VII Hospital Sanatorium, but this was specifically for the transport of infectious cases.

The first motorised ambulance

It might be expected that the conversion from horse-drawn to motorised transport in 1926 would be a notable event, but it was afforded little significance in the recollections of Mr. Davidson, son of the future Master and Matron of the Hospital. He later recalled with stark simplicity: *"they bought a lorry chassis, took the body off the horse ambulance and bolted it to the Bean chassis."*

It is of interest to note that no such conversion took place at the King Edward Sanatorium, which purchased a new automobile ambulance for infectious cases in 1929 at a cost of £430.

For the first part of the century the conversion to motorised transport was the only significant progress in the provision of ambulance services to the island. The ambulance service remained a vehicle, for getting prostrate bodies to the hospital. It did not carry equipment with which to perform treatment, and to drive it you needed a road licence, not first aid or medical training.

One of those licenced to drive the new motorised vehicle was Joe Way, who owned a garage in the Pollet. When the ambulance was needed the doctor or the Master of the Town Hospital would telephone Joe Way at his garage. As Mr. Davidson junior recalls, *"Basil Harwood and Cliff Davison were his mechanics. When you wanted the ambulance to go out you phoned Joe Way and he or one of his mechanics would come up. He would come, and an inmate would go with him to handle the other end of the stretcher."*

The use of an inmate from the Poor Law institution to act as attendant on the ambulance is also recalled by Reginald Blanchford, who was later to have a dramatic effect on the Island's ambulance service. He remembers seeing the ambulance arrive with a member of the poor house who had been called away from his lunch, and who still had the egg or soup splashes running down his front when he arrived to take a patient to hospital.

Although this may seem like a remarkably low standard, it was accepted practice, and mirrored the situation in most of the UK, where the ambulance was also just a means of transport, perhaps operated by a miners' lodge or a friendly society.

Mr Way also had a job for a time as part-time fireman, and was sometimes away from his garage. When the ambulance was needed he had to be contacted to return to the hospital, take the ambulance out of its garage next to the mortuary, pick up an attendant, and then drive to the incident. Calling out the ambulance was therefore not a quick operation, and it was this fact which led to a major change in the ambulance service in Guernsey.

Reginald Blanchford's vision

In a hit and run accident during a rainstorm one night in 1930, a taxi cab collided with a motorcycle, sending the teenage rider crashing into a wall. The cab did not stop.

The motorcyclist was found unconscious, covered in blood and rain and hardly breathing, by a schoolteacher called Frank le Poidevin. He realised that by the time he had telephoned for the ambulance and it eventually arrived with its untrained crew, it would simply be needed to convey a dead body.

A passing motorist stopped to help in his two-seater convertible. Mr Ulric Ash, of Ash's Garages, helped Mr le Poidevin into the passenger's seat, with the lifeless motorcyclist on top of him, advised him to hook his foot round the door as the patient's broken leg was hanging out, and drove through the rain to the Victoria Cottage Hospital at Amherst.

That motorcyclist was Reginald Blanchford, a teenager who was having difficulty settling into a job after leaving school. He remained unconscious for eight days, with multiple injuries including a broken skull, jaw, ribs, pelvis, thigh, leg and ankle. The ambulance was never called.

Four years later he was still receiving treatment as a result of his injuries when he learned that the St John Ambulance Brigade had been formed in Guernsey. This news gave him a purpose in life which some would say became an obsession. He reasoned that he would not still be suffering from the effects of his injuries, if at the time of his accident an ambulance had been more readily available, staffed by people trained in first aid, like the Brigade members. The St John Ambulance Brigade could provide a means by which he could improve the service given to other accident victims.

He enrolled in the division as a private, and with as much diplomacy as could be expected of an enthusiastic nineteen-year-old on a mission, began suggesting that the division could be of great service to the community if it bought an ambulance.

Some could see nothing wrong with the Town Hospital service which had served the island for years, but others could see the potential. Jurat John Rousell, who was vice president of the Division, put up £100 to buy a second-hand Talbot ambulance from the UK, and avoluntary contribution scheme was started to raise the funds to maintain it.

Jurat Rousell made his contribution, advocating *"a careful and modest start in this new venture"*.

Private Blanchford had studied anatomy and physiology during his recuperation, whilst gaining qualifications in massage and medical electricity, and he offered to act as unpaid driver of the vehicle. When the black Talbot arrived in late May 1936 it was parked in a purpose-built garage in the grounds of his father's concrete works in the Rohais, just outside St Peter Port.

Word soon spread that an alternative ambulance to that of the Town Hospital had been set up, and by the end of July 1936 the ambulance contribution scheme was progressing satisfactorily and the ambulance was being used about once each day.

This embryonic ambulance service was known as the Transport Section of the St John Ambulance Brigade, to distinguish it from the other activities of the division, such as supplying volunteer first aiders to attend cinema shows and other gatherings.

Volunteer Brigade members assisted full-time driver Blanchford in providing 24 hour cover, and when time allowed, a member from the new female division was called, since they were trained in home nursing.

After just one year, in June 1937, the full-time staff rose to two, and at the end of the year confidence was such that advertisements were circulated advising: *"For Ambulance - ring 70"*.

Not surprisingly, the Town Hospital service took exception to the new pretender, with its implication that the official, States-run ambulance had deficiencies. The rivalry became bitter, on some occasions both vehicles arriving at the same accident scene. The St John Brigade even made representations to the President of the Poor Law Board when a St John ambulance scheme contributor was forced to use the Town ambulance!

The main advantage of the new St John Transport Section, however, was that it had a full-time driver who was immediately available, and staff trained in first aid, two important features which the Town ambulance could not match.

As time went by, doctors and others began to accept the new service, and in 1939 a formal proposal was made by Brigade Surgeon Dr W.B. Fox for the Brigade to take over the whole of the Island's ambulance transport, except for the infectious cases of the King Edward Hospital service. This was put to the States of Guernsey in the form of a requete from Jurat John Rousell, which was approved in December of that year. It included a provision for the States to replace the ambulance vehicles when necessary, and gave a grant of £200 per year to assist with its work.

The War Years

The year 1939 was not a good time to start anything new, of course, and the realities of war struck Guernsey with a vengeance in the June of the following year. In three days a voluntary evacuation of the Island saw 23,000 islanders leave for the UK, and the St John Transport section, now the official Island ambulance service, assisted with the transport of many infirm and sick residents from homes to the docks.

Later that month on 28 June, came the air raid which killed 30 islanders. A Brigade ambulance was severely damaged and in a cruel twist of fate carried one of the fatally wounded casualties, Joe Way.

The Service continued during the war, providing an efficient and comprehensive service which, despite the inevitable shortages of food, petrol and other provisions, was able to report that no call went unanswered. Blanchford was later to describe the work during the occupation as the "Service's finest hour".

Members were initially refused permission to wear any form of uniform, but the St John Ambulance Brigade gradually became a focal group for welfare work among the population, in the latter years being charged with guarding and distributing the precious Red Cross parcels which arrived by ship.

Post war progress

When the war ended Blanchford's father sold his Rohais site to the Brigade and a new ambulance station was built. Staff increased to four ambulancemen and a paid secretary who, as a female St John member, also doubled as a nurse ambulance attendant when necessary.

The war had seen a great improvement in the fields of electronics and radio technology, and in 1947 Guernsey's service became the first ambulance service in the British Isles to install two-way mobile radios.

In 1952, an application was made to the States for funds to buy a new ambulance to replace the one bought in 1938, and a typical compromise saw the service given the more modern vehicle of the King Edward Hospital, on condition that it also took on responsibility for the transport of infectious cases. The service thus became responsible for all ambulance work in the island.

That same year saw the inauguration of the world's first dedicated ambulance launch. This idea was born out of the frustration experienced when the service was called to offshore incidents. The delay whilst the ambulance staff tried to find a boat and skipper who could ferry them to a casualty, who might be badly injured on offshore rocks at the base of cliffs, or even on the other islands of Herm or Sark, was frustrating for the staff and sometimes serious for the patient.

The problem was resolved in 1952 when the ferry *Flying Christine* was bought from local skipper Don le Prevost, equipped inside like a road ambulance, and moored permanently available in St Peter Port harbour. Don le Prevost offered his services as unpaid coxswain to the ambulance service, and was soon joined by other honorary coxswains, and in its first year the launch performed over 20 missions.

Many developments grew from seeds which had been sown during the Occupation. Records kept during the war developed into a formal blood donor register held at the ambulance station. When donors were required, the hospital called the ambulance service, which contacted suitable donors, offered transport if needed, and maintained an up-to-date record of attendance. This continued until 1986, when the activity was transferred to the more logical responsibility of the hospital pathology department.

When civilian flights between Guernsey and the UK resumed after the Occupation, the service established arrangements with the airlines for patients who needed to travel to the UK for treatment. This developed into a highly organised operation, which in emergencies could charter aircraft and open airports within an hour, and by the end of the century the service was arranging an average of 300 journeys a year to almost any destination.

In the days before the war, a small hut had been incorporated at Blanchford's father's concrete works for callers with minor injuries who wanted advice from the Brigade's first aiders. When the ambulance station was expanded after the Occupation, two dedicated rooms were built, where patients with minor injuries could be examined by the paid staff on standby, and either be treated or referred to a doctor. By the late eighties almost 4000 patients a year were taking advantage of this free service.

The *Flying Christine* was frequently despatched to rescue casualties on rocks or at the base of cliffs, and on such occasions the crew used a rubber dinghy from the launch to reach close inshore. Efforts to improve safety and minimise the aggravation of patients' injuries led to improved designs, and in 1961 the service introduced the island's first powered inflatable inshore rescue boat.

In a similar way casualties from cliffs were rescued by ambulancemen with ropes and pulleys, and by the nineteen seventies this had developed into a specialised team, with members of the paid staff training with mountain rescue teams in the UK.

Much of the expansion in rescue and ancillary activities was a result of Reginald Blanchford's insatiable desire to provide the best service possible, and his untiring pursuit of sponsors to help the cause. The service was part of a charitable organisation: although it received a grant from the States to help with the costs of the road ambulances, it was not States-owned. It therefore had the freedom to establish or expand services if it could find donors willing to fund the activities, and many individuals, charities and societies helped to raise funds as they saw the value of the services it provided.

One very generous benefactor was the Hayward Foundation, set up by Sir Charles Hayward, one-time resident of the isle of Jethou. This foundation paid for an electronic indicator which automatically updated the location of ambulances on a map in the control room using radio signals sent from the vehicles themselves. Installed in 1969, this was featured on the television programme "Tomorrow's World" and pre dated by some 20 years the spread of vehicle tracking in UK services, based on global positioning satellite technology.

The Hayward foundation also purchased the island's first breeches-buoy for the service, and in 1969 funded a portable one-man recompression chamber. This was followed in 1973 by a static ten-man chamber, the first such recompression centre in the British Isles in civilian hands, installed in its own purpose-built room at the ambulance station. With its own staff trained to operate the chamber, and also manning the ambulances and the ambulance launch, the service was able to give an unbeatable speed of response to divers in difficulties.

Perhaps the most technically advanced project financed by the Hayward foundation was a mobile radar unit. The first of its kind in the world, this was developed by Decca and towed from the ambulance station to a number of predetermined locations around the island. With Home Office approval this was used to test the use of transponders at sea by the lifeboat and marine ambulance in the early seventies.

With its wide range of activities Guernsey's service became recognised and highly respected as a combined ambulance and rescue organisation. Ambulance staff maintained hydraulic cutting equipment to release trapped patients from vehicles or machinery, together with breathing apparatus, and even incorporated a sub-aqua diving team into the service's response.

As the demands on the service grew, the number of full-time staff increased. Inevitably the reliance on voluntary Brigade members decreased, and by the early seventies the ambulances were crewed exclusively by paid full-time staff, who wore a modified uniform introduced in 1968.

This indicated their rank in the service, now known as the Ambulance & Rescue Service, from any other Brigade rank, for permanent staff were still expected to belong to one of the voluntary St John Ambulance Brigade divisions, which involved regular first aid training evenings, attending an annual inspection, and passing an annual examination in first aid.

Reg Blanchford resigns

It did not escape the notice of many staff that they were more highly trained than their Brigade officers, and that overtime hours to cope with the demands of the service were deemed to be part of voluntary duties and were therefore unpaid.

This situation was unique among ambulance staff, for the St John Ambulance Brigade and other agencies had ceased to provide statutory emergency ambulance services in the UK. Local government changes of 1974 placed all ambulance services within the National Health Service, so Guernsey was the only place in the British Isles where the ambulance service was run by St John.

This led to major upset when a St John Commander was appointed in Guernsey. This rank was normally responsible for all St John activities in any area, but uniquely in Guernsey these activities included a professional ambulance service. Reg Blanchford saw this as equivalent to placing the head of the special constabulary in charge of the regular Police force, and resigned in protest.

The resignation of the man who was acknowledged as the founder of the St John Ambulance & Rescue Service, was seen by some as the end of an era, by others as the end of the service, but his parting message to his staff was to carry on rendering the service to the public in the way he had taught them.

The service continued under Ronald Herve, who was being trained to be the next Chief Officer. During his term of office, a medical comforts store run by the service was converted into a large showroom hiring and selling aids for the disabled, and non operational staff were recruited specifically for this service. This grew into the largest centre for such equipment in the Channel Islands, and proved to be of great value to community nurses and those looking after patients who lived at home.

With the elderly population increasing and more people being cared for at home, there was a growth in the number who needed regular visits to out-patient or therapy departments. A second tier of ambulance staff was created in 1983, employed on day time shifts only, trained specifically in the ambulance transport needs of such patients rather than in the whole range of emergency duties.

It was this tier which attracted the service's first female ambulance member, who later went on to the front-line service, laying the foundation for future female practitioners and paramedics.

Unwelcome changes

A new Board of Management had been formed following Blanchford's resignation, with an independent chairman rather than a St John officer at its head, and the service underwent several reviews. One of the most influential took place in 1984, when a Chief Ambulance Officer from the UK argued that Guernsey's ambulance staff could not keep up with the training needed to stay proficient in all the rescue and ambulance activities of the service, and embarked on a series of drastic cuts.

Without ceremony the mobile radar unit was de-commissioned, the rescue trailer dismantled, and the sub-aqua diving team disbanded. Even the possibility of closing the first aid room, and scrapping the cliff rescue team, inshore rescue boats and marine ambulance was considered, but later rejected.

Perhaps the most important recommendation for the future, however, was the decision that a St John first aid certificate was no longer sufficient qualification for staff who worked in an emergency ambulance service.

New training standards had been laid down for NHS ambulance staff in the UK, in what was known as Ambulance Aid. Guernsey's personnel also trained to these standards, but could not receive formal certification since they were trained and tested outside the United Kingdom. On paper, therefore, the only recognised certificates held by the staff were St John Ambulance first aid certificates.

The decision was taken that training at an NHS accredited ambulance centre in the UK would be a minimum for Guernsey's staff, who would no longer pursue St John Ambulance qualifications.

The severity of the 1984 review took its toll of the Chief Officer, who resigned in that year. A new head, Michael Dene, was appointed in 1985. He had joined as a private under Reginald Blanchford, and after a five year tenure in which to implement the review's recommendations and stabilise the service, he became the first chief officer to retire normally in 1990.

Paramedic skills and the future

His successor, Neil Tucker, took over at a time when ambulance services were emerging as a potential front-line of emergency medicine. It was being realised that ambulance staff could be trained in some techniques, formerly the prerogative of doctors in hospital, which could significantly improve patients' conditions, or even survival, if applied at the scene of an accident.

For some years the service had carried one defibrillator for doctors' use, but in 1990 defibrillators were installed on all front-line ambulances and staff began training in their use. When advances in technology produced a new generation of defibrillators in 1997, the Service became the first in the British Isles to equip all its vehicles, including non-emergency vehicles, with defibrillation capability.

A standard range of advanced skills became known as ambulance paramedic skills. These required extra training in the UK followed by practical experience under doctors in operating theatres. An application to the Board of Health for an increase in the grant to allow the introduction of paramedic training in Guernsey was rejected, but Tucker persuaded his Board of Management to trial the idea, and in 1992 the service's training officer, Jon Beausire, became the island's first ambulance paramedic. By the end of the decade the 'trial' was continuing, with 24-hour cover provided by 11 ambulance paramedics.

New skills were incorporated into training for all staff, and in 1996 following a review of major incident procedures, a voluntary ambulance reserve was established. This consisted of volunteers trained to assist the service in a range of tasks needed at a major accident, rather than just to provide first aid, so that ambulance staff could be free to apply improved patient care.

Neil Tucker, who had been recruited by Reg Blanchford, took the view that the improvement in staff capability together with their rescue activities gave the public of Guernsey a formidable combination. Trapped or injured casualties were rescued by personnel able to assess and treat injuries with the skill of professional ambulance staff, who could then arrange evacuation in full consideration of the patients' clinical needs.

As the century drew to a close, the St John Ambulance organisation in England underwent a major restructuring exercise, in an attempt to adapt to changing times. To protect Guernsey's unique service, the Ambulance & Rescue Service was formally constituted as a company limited by guarantee in 1999.

In the same year, an Act of Parliament in the UK introduced the State Registration of paramedics, to include those in Guernsey's service. In a way this was official recognition that the skills of ambulance staff now extended into professional medicine, and even included techniques which some doctors would hesitate to perform outside a hospital setting.

The horse and cart of the Town Hospital seem a hundred years away.....

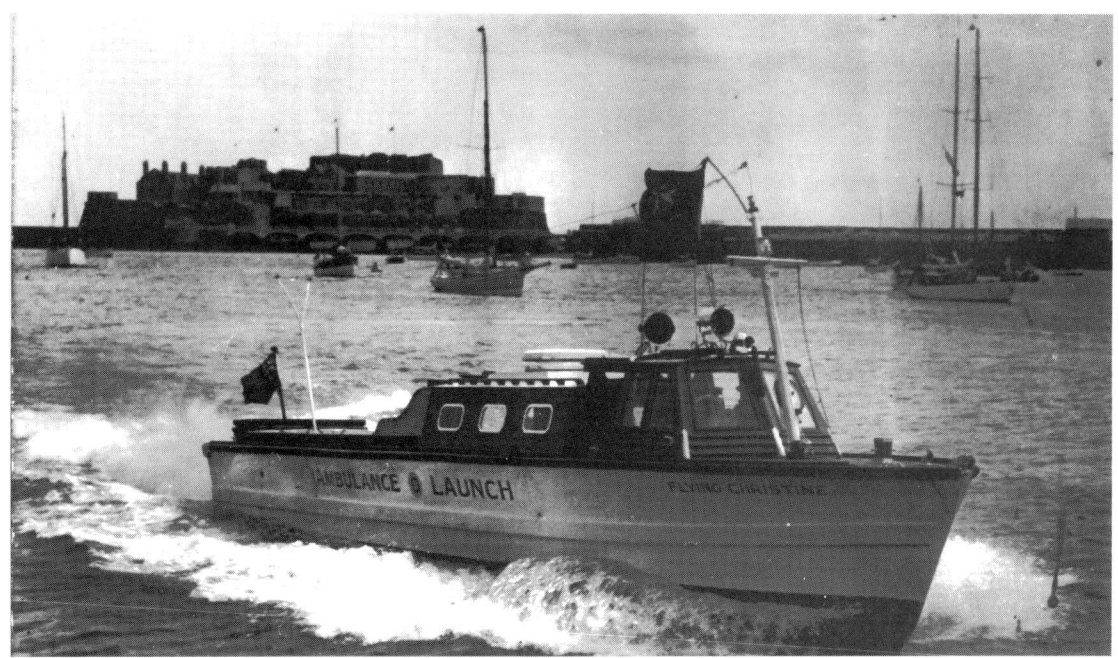

Ambulance launch - Flying Christine I

'1952 saw the inauguration of the world's first dedicated ambulance launch, when the ferry Flying Christine was bought from local skipper Don le Prevost, equipped inside like a road ambulance, and moored permanently available in St Peter Port harbour ...... in its first year the launch performed over 20 missions.' (Chapter Fourteen)

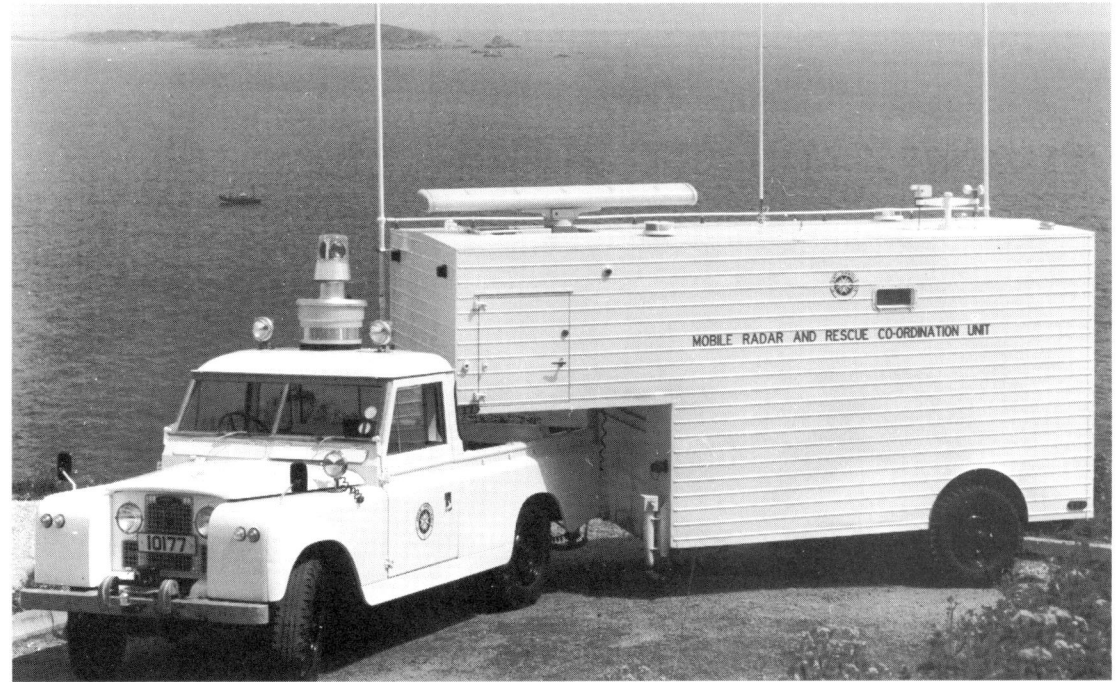

Radar Unit

'Perhaps the most technically advanced project financed by the Hayward Foundation was a mobile radar unit. It was the first of its kind in the world ....' (Chapter Fourteen)

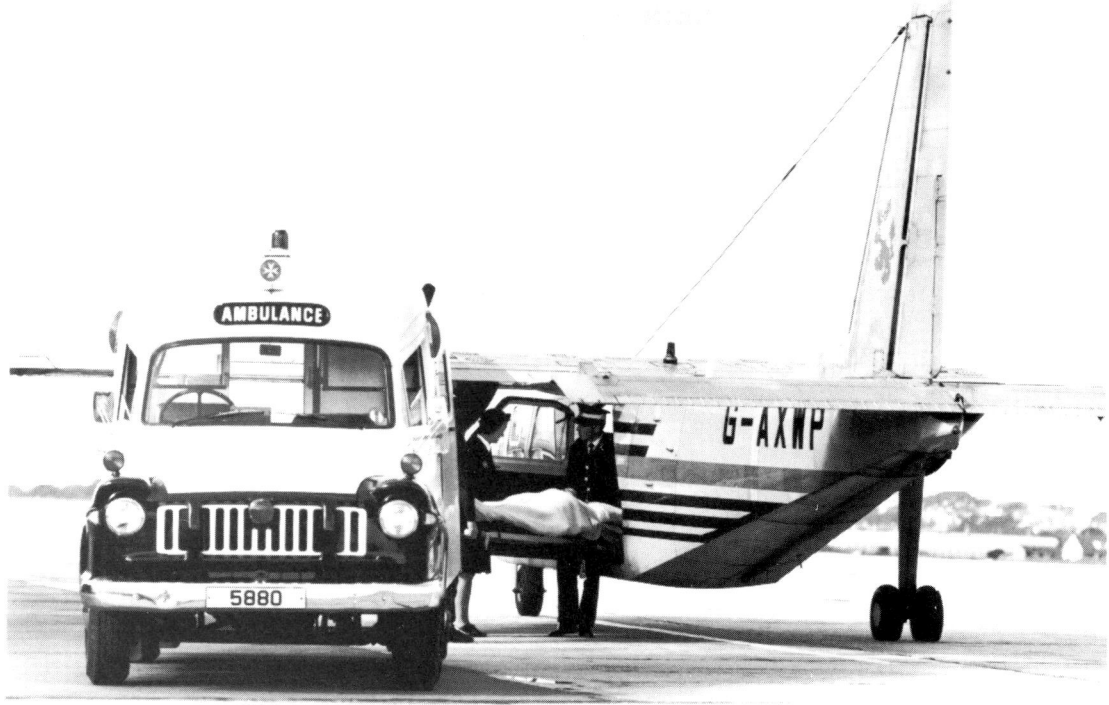

Air Charter

'The service established arrangements with the airlines for patients who needed to travel to the UK for treatment ...... by the end of the century the service was arranging an average of 300 journeys a year to almost any destination'. (Chapter Fourteen)

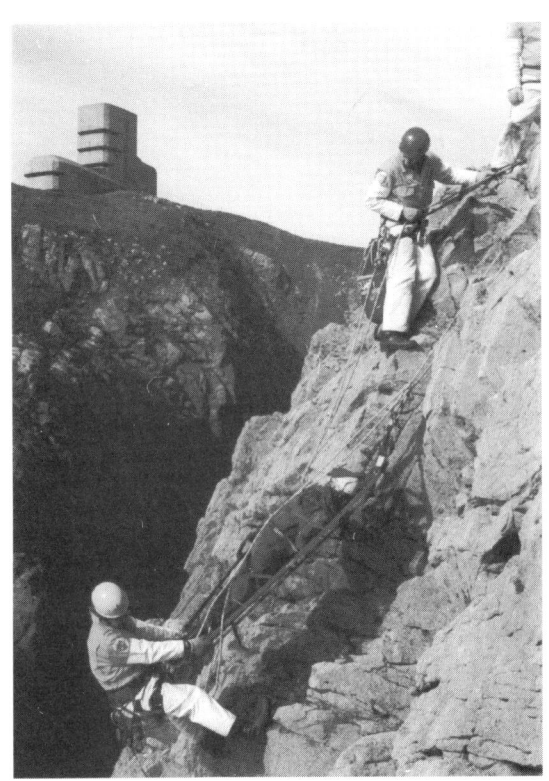

Cliff Rescue

'The improvement in staff capability together with their rescue activities gave the public of Guernsey a formidable combination. Trapped or injured casualties were rescued by personnel able to assess and treat injuries with the skill of professional ambulance staff' (Chapter Fourteen)

Chapter Fifteen

Health Care in Alderney

Philip Cranford-Smith

The Board of Health's mandate requires that it "maintain and improve the health of the people of Guernsey and Alderney.........'. The history of health in the northern isle has of necessity taken a somewhat different course to the paths in Guernsey, but increasingly since the involvement of the Board of Health in 1948, the separate paths are now converging.

The Reverend Mignot's Legacy

Apart from periods in the latter part of the nineteenth and early part of the twentieth centuries when detachments of the British Army were garrisoned on the island and their field hospital may have been available to care for civilian emergencies, Alderney was without a hospital altogether until the 1920s. There was no place where a patient who was seriously ill could receive attention and nursing, apart from their own home. Unlike today, home confinements were, of necessity, the rule rather than the exception. Accidents in the island's main industry of quarrying, and in the harbour were quite frequent.

Connection with Guernsey was by sea, and during the winter months the steamer sailed but twice weekly. In these circumstances it was often necessary for patients who needed urgent medical treatment to be sent to Guernsey by open boat, at times in appallingly bad weather. Such transport did not improve the patient's chance of survival and a trying journey was not unknown to have fatal results.

In the early 1920s a number of public spirited residents were moved to try and remedy this unsatisfactory state of affairs, and a start was made in organising a public subscription with a view to providing a first aid ward where initial treatment and skilled nursing could be provided until such time as the patient could be moved to a Guernsey hospital by the steamer.

The Reverend Peter Mignot, an Alderney Parson living in Guernsey, became interested in the project and came to Alderney for discussions with the local Committee. The outcome of this meeting was an offer by Rev. Mignot to purchase a suitable property and transfer its title in trust into the names of members of the Committee who would become the first Trustees. He furthermore offered to provide the necessary furnishings and to establish a modest endowment towards the running costs. All this was to be as a memorial to his first wife.

Although there were some at the time who felt that the Rev. Mignot's offer went far beyond the original ideas, his generous offer was gratefully accepted by the Committee, and on 23 June 1925 the Victoria Hotel at 55 Victoria Street was purchased by the trustees (Rev. Mignot being one of their number) for the sum of £1000. This building would provide accommodation for seven or eight patients and included a basic operating theatre.

A voluntary committee was formed to take on the management of the new hospital which was to be named the Mignot Memorial Hospital, and over the years preceding the evacuation of the population in 1940, it did splendid work in raising funds to supplement the small charges which were all that most patients could afford. Whist drives, dances, pound days, concerts and door to door collections all helped the hospital to pay its way, augmented from time to time by generous donations from the Reverend Mignot's widow. For several years the States of Alderney voted a grant of £50 towards the hospital funds.

Full use was made of the facilities offered by the new hospital and the local doctors much appreciated the opportunity to provide their patients with skilled nursing. On more than one occasion urgent surgical operations were performed, the doctors co-operating, generally with success.(!)

Evacuation, Occupation and after

In 1940 the whole population was evacuated and the island occupied by German military forces. Although the occupying forces built a large fortified bunker type hospital at Longis Road, it appears that they also continued to use the Mignot as a hospital, and on the return of the islanders in 1945 a certain amount of furnishings and German surgical equipment remained. Whatever was of use was retained and the hospital was re-equipped with the aid of H M Government. In 1974 a collection of German instruments were rediscovered in the loft of the new Mignot Memorial Hospital. (p.163)

The German forces had established a dental centre in the basement of the hospital and this was retained and used at regular intervals by a visiting Dental Surgeon from Guernsey until the eventual arrival of a resident Dental Surgeon. In the early months of 1946, as the islanders were gradually returning, a number of prisoners of war were kept on the island to assist with the repairs and renovations which were needed. During this time a number of islanders benefited from treatment from the German military surgeon and dentist who were among the prisoners.

With the general rise in costs following the war, it was soon apparent that the Mignot Hospital could not continue to serve its useful purpose on the initial voluntary funding without further financial aid, and a request to the States of Alderney for a larger grant received sympathetic consideration, enabling the hospital to balance its budget.

In 1947, following concern on the part of H M Government as to the viability of an independent Alderney, a Committee of the Privy Council carried out an enquiry into the state of the island, with particular reference to its form of government and its relationship with the neighbouring islands, its financial position and its economic prospects.

As a result of this enquiry and its recommendations, an agreement was reached between Alderney and Guernsey on the transfer to Guernsey of administrative and financial responsibility for a number of subjects, one of which was Health Services. This transfer of functions took place on 1 January 1949 under "*The Alderney (Application of Legislation) Law 1948*". This is generally referred to as the "1948 agreement".

Thus the Board of Health became responsible for all matters relating to public health in Alderney, a subject that had hitherto received scant attention. The resident medical practitioner was appointed as Deputy Medical Officer of Health with responsibility for Public Health in Alderney, and the services of officers of the Board became available to carry out inspections and give advice as they do at present.

Perhaps somewhat surprisingly for a committee appointed by a Labour government, only passing reference was made to the hospital service in Alderney and no recommendations made. The Mignot Memorial Hospital therefore continued to function on a voluntary basis, administered by a lay Committee and assisted by an annual grant from the States of Alderney. The Jubilee Home, established as a workhouse in 1887, remained under the control of the States of Alderney as a residential home for the elderly. No nursing care was provided at the Jubilee.

At this time the island was served by one physician and three nurses, one of whom was part time, but it was becoming apparent, in the light of modern thought and advances in medical treatment and nursing, that the existing building and service had become increasingly unsuitable. In addition the building was old, not designed as a hospital, and costly to maintain. Although it was clear that a completely new hospital was needed, the Management Committee did not feel, in view of the then uncertain state of the island's finances, that the States could be asked to fund this.

After researching various possibilities, the Committee approached the Nuffield Provincial Hospitals Trust, in the hope that some assistance might be forthcoming.

It seems that the application to the Nuffield Trust was made at a most opportune time, and after discussion and visits from L Farrer-Brown, its Honorary Secretary, the Trust agreed that the existing building was most unsuitable and had outlived its purpose.

The Trust had the vision to imagine a Health Centre concept and agreed a grant of £20,000, later increased by £2,000, to build and establish a new hospital, providing the States of Alderney were prepared to guarantee sufficient funds for the efficient maintenance of the new building.

Various sites for the new hospital were suggested and inspected. The one most favoured was that overlooking Crabby Bay, owned by Rowe and Mitchell Ltd, who had been part of the pre-war quarrying industry.

Mr F L Impey, one of the founders of Kalamazoo Ltd the well known business stationery company, had been a regular visitor to Alderney since the 1930s and had retired to the island in 1946 having purchased Fort Corblets. He served as a member of the States of Alderney from 1949 to 1957. He had done much to re-establish the economy after the war, giving much needed employment in the conversion of his Fort into luxury accommodation, and had set up a horticultural research station and market gardening enterprise. He now decided to purchase the Crabby site and presented it as a philanthropic gift to the island. This land was to be held in the name of the Hospital Trustees, who on completion of the new building would sell the Victoria Street property.

Mr Impey was later to contribute substantially towards the furnishing and equipping of the new hospital.

The Mignot Memorial Hospital reborn

Plans for the new building were prepared under the direction of R Llewelyn Davies, Head of the Nuffield Foundation for Architectural Studies, and the contract for the construction placed with a local company. The unusual design consisted of a number of linked units with steeply pitched roofs, the whole building being faced with stone reclaimed from the demolition of the nearby Roman Catholic church which had been damaged beyond viable repair during the German occupation. It has to be said that there were at the time some local misgivings as to the practicality of the design, which it was felt was overcomplicated, and was unkindly likened by some as looking like a collection of cowsheds, but of course the Committee would have found it extremely difficult to question such a generous gift. Time has however borne out some of those misgivings, as it has been difficult to plan extensions to the original building in an efficient manner. As a result the building of today has a disjointed layout and is more difficult to staff and maintain than would have been the case had the original layout taken possible future expansion into account.

The new building consisted of two three-bedded wards and two single wards opening out onto a dayroom with access to bathrooms and toilets. There was an operating theatre and out-patients clinic and three staff bedrooms were integral with the building.

On 27 July 1957 the foundation stone was laid by Her Majesty Queen Elizabeth II who, accompanied by HRH Prince Philip had arrived in the Royal Yacht Britannia. The silver trowel used by Her Majesty in this ceremony may be seen in the entrance hall of the Court House.

The new hospital opened in 1958 and the Trustees sold 55 Victoria Street, investing the proceeds for the benefit of the new hospital which took the name of its predecessor.

At this time, as the States had guaranteed funding it was agreed that the constitution of the Management Committee should be redrawn. It would now include three States members, one of whom would be Chairman, the States Treasurer, ex officio, an Honorary Secretary and three ordinary members elected by the public and the Deputy Medical Officer of Health.

After only a few years of operation it became clear that staffing levels required were considerably in excess of the four originally estimated, and insufficient staff accommodation had been provided. However, thanks to a most generous donation from Brigadier F G French, who had been Judge of Alderney from 1938 to 1946, a Matron's bungalow with an additional staff bedroom and laundry room was built adjacent to the hospital and completed in 1960. This was named "The Anne French Annexe" in memory of the benefactor's late wife. Brigadier French also set up a trust fund for the maintenance of the building.

Need for expansion

During the early 1960s, as Alderney returned to normality after the war time desecration, the population steadily grew, thanks to a mini-building boom. Many of the new settlers were at or near retirement age, a fact which would later lead to the need for greater provision for long term care, both residential and nursing.

By the end of the 1960s this pressure was starting to be felt, with many of the hospital beds being taken up by long stay beds, often necessitating the use of overflow beds in the day room area. At this time most confinements were still taking place in Alderney, and concerns were raised by the Committee's medical advisers about the dangers of mixing maternity patients with general cases.

The committee came to the conclusion that to solve this problem a new maternity wing should be built and plans were drawn up for an extension on the North side of the hospital. This would provide one three-bedded ward and one single ward, together with a milk kitchen, bathroom, toilets and sluice. The connecting corridor would provide an additional room which would later become the X-ray department.

These proposals were put to the States of Alderney, which on 27 February 1969 agreed to fund the construction of the new wing. The initial cost was estimated to be £19,000, but due to the lowest tender being withdrawn, plus additional unexpected foundation works, the final cost was £24,000. A grant of £4,500 towards furnishings and equipment was received from the Mason Trust in the UK, in recognition of which the extension was named the Mason Wing. The new wing was completed and opened in 1970.

In spite of the extra accommodation provided by the Mason Wing, the introduction of a district nursing service in 1972, and extensions to the residential accommodation at the Jubilee Home in 1973, pressure for long stay beds continued to mount and it became clear by the mid 1970s that extra accommodation was urgently needed. However, because the States funds for capital projects were limited it was also clear that the cost of a traditionally built extension would not be acceptable and the Committee had to consider alternatives.

The advice of the Board of Health was sought and the Committee was told that the Board had itself faced similar problems of shortages of accommodation and had decided to use a prefabricated wooden building, supplied by the Guernsey firm of F A Falla, as a short term solution. The expected life of such a building was about twenty-five years.

Having inspected this building in Guernsey, the Committee had plans drawn up for a new long stay wing, containing two wards of six beds each, together with bathroom and toilet facilities and a dayroom. The estimated cost of supply and construction was £27,300 and funds were voted for the new wing by the States on 23 January 1974.

The wing was ready for occupation before the end of the year and officially opened by Mrs Margery Baron, wife of the President, and named "The Aurigny Wing" on 31 December 1974.

The Board of Health takes over ....

At the beginning of the 1970s the increasing complexities of running a modern hospital led the Management Committee to approach the Board of Health with the aim of some assistance in running it. It was also thought that economies could be achieved by taking advantage of the Board's greater purchasing power, and by making use of its technical services. At about the same time public pressure was being applied on the States for 'free' beds to be made available at the Mignot as had been introduced in Guernsey in 1973.

After many meetings and much discussion the outcome was a recommendation which was accepted by both States that the administration of the hospital should be taken over by the Board of Health with effect from 1 January 1975 to be operated and financed as a 'transferred service' in the same manner as those other services, including Public Health, which had been operated by Guernsey since 1949. As a consequence of this transfer beds in both the Mignot and the Princess Elizabeth Hospital became free of charge to the patient, except for long stay patients who continued to be charged according to means.

The Management Committee continued in being for a while but was soon disbanded and liaison established between the Board and the Alderney Health and Welfare Committee. The Trustees of course continued to own the land and all the buildings which had been erected on it, but the income from its investments was only sufficient to pay the annual owners rates.

In addition, a fine new Day-Room, the Alice May Buckle Room, had been constructed with magnificent views to the North and in which patients may sit or walk around.

In 1974, the final year under the old regime, a States grant of £39,900 had been necessary.

The X-ray equipment at the Mignot had been installed in 1969 at his own expense by Mr Graham Lawson a local radiographer.

The Board considered this to be a rather unsatisfactory situation and one of its first acts was the purchase of the equipment, with Mr Lawson becoming an employee of the Board. Since that time the X-ray equipment has been upgraded and in 1997 the department obtained an ultrasound scanner, thanks to a generous legacy to the League of Friends from the late Mrs Nancy Norton.

With the opening of the Aurigny Wing the number of beds doubled, from 12 to 24, and although the Management Committee had rather optimistically predicted that no extra staff would be needed, it soon became apparent that more staff were required. Whenever possible locally resident staff were recruited, but there were insufficient trained nurses to fill all posts and nurses were brought in from the UK and Ireland. The original staff accommodation and bungalow was insufficient and it became necessary to rent a house in St Anne's for additional staff accommodation. This was a far from satisfactory solution, and in 1981 the States of Alderney agreed to the building of six nurses flatlets on land near the hospital. Each flatlet was centrally heated and contained a bed-sitting room, kitchen and bathroom. There was a communal laundry facility. It was the opinion of the Health and Welfare Committee at the time that accommodation of a high standard was necessary in order to retain staff, and the flatlets compare very favourably with staff accommodation elsewhere.

Since 1993 the Matron has been locally resident, providing the opportunity to make alternative use of the Anne French Annexe. The lounge and one other room are used as a consulting room and waiting room by Health Visitors, Ophthalmologists, Paediatrician and other visiting specialists; also as a meeting and lecture room; the remainder of the building provides much needed storage space.

In 1980 a major project to renew all heating and electrical services and construct a separate services block to include boiler house, incinerator and laundry was carried out. At the same time the mortuary was upgraded.

Mention must be made of the invaluable work of the hospital's League of Friends who apart from the regular visits to attend to flowers and patient's trolley, have over the years raised considerable funds for equipment and capital projects. These include the sun lounge, with its superb sea view, a relatives room, a patio and gazebo, the first district nurses' car and many other items.

The improved services at the hospital, with regular visits by visiting specialists and the extension of the district nursing service mean that the concept of a 'medical centre' envisaged by the Nuffield Foundation has come to fruition.

Latterly, the advantages of closer relationships between the islands, as demonstrated by that provided by the Board of Health, have resulted in improved health care beyond all recognition. This has been heavily underlined by the ready access to the Princess Elizabeth Hospital for Alderney people in all aspects of a modern health service but, in particular, the care for expectant mothers as well as accident and emergency treatment.

It should be emphasised that none of the latter could be achievable without the willing assistance of the local airline, St John Ambulance and all associated with both airports.

Comparison with the state of affairs before 1925 as described in the first paragraphs serves to highlight the enormous advances in health care, public health and communications over the last three-quarters of a century and particularly the last 25 years. The population of the 1920s would find it unrecognisable now.

The above article has been compiled with the most appreciated assistance of Mr John Sumner, who has supplied a great deal of additional information.

Acknowledgements are also due to Mr Brian Bonnard for the use of the photograph of the original Mignot Hospital in Victoria Street.

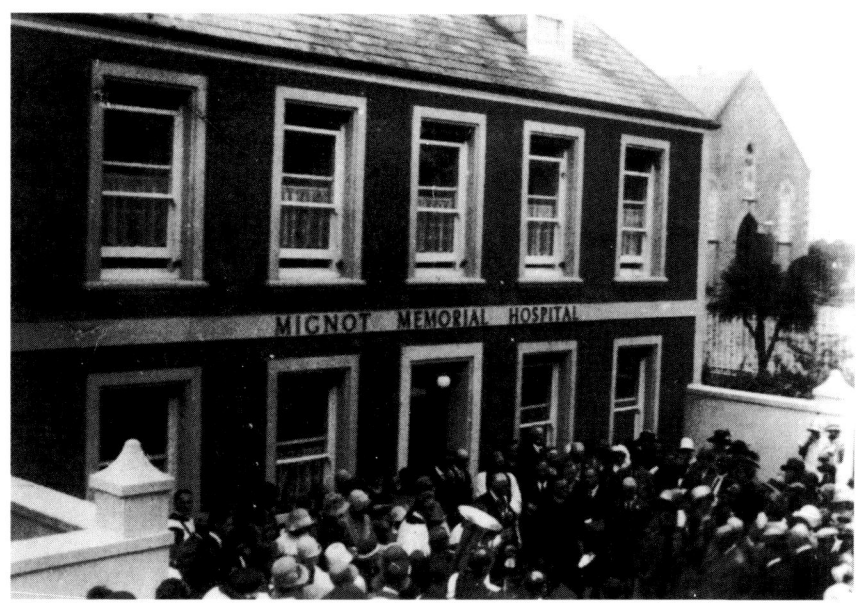

Opening of the original Mignot Memorial Hospital, St. Anne's, Alderney

'On 23rd June 1925 the Victoria Hotel at 55, Victoria Street was purchased by the trustees (Rev. Mignot being one of their number) for the sum of £1000.' (Chapter Fifteen)

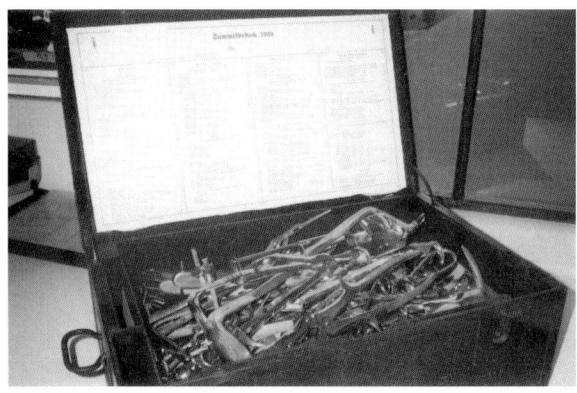

"*In 1974, a collection of German instruments were rediscovered in the loft of the new Mignot Memorial Hospital*". (Chapter Fifteen). These instruments may currently be viewed in the Alderney Society Musueum, St Anne's, Alderney.

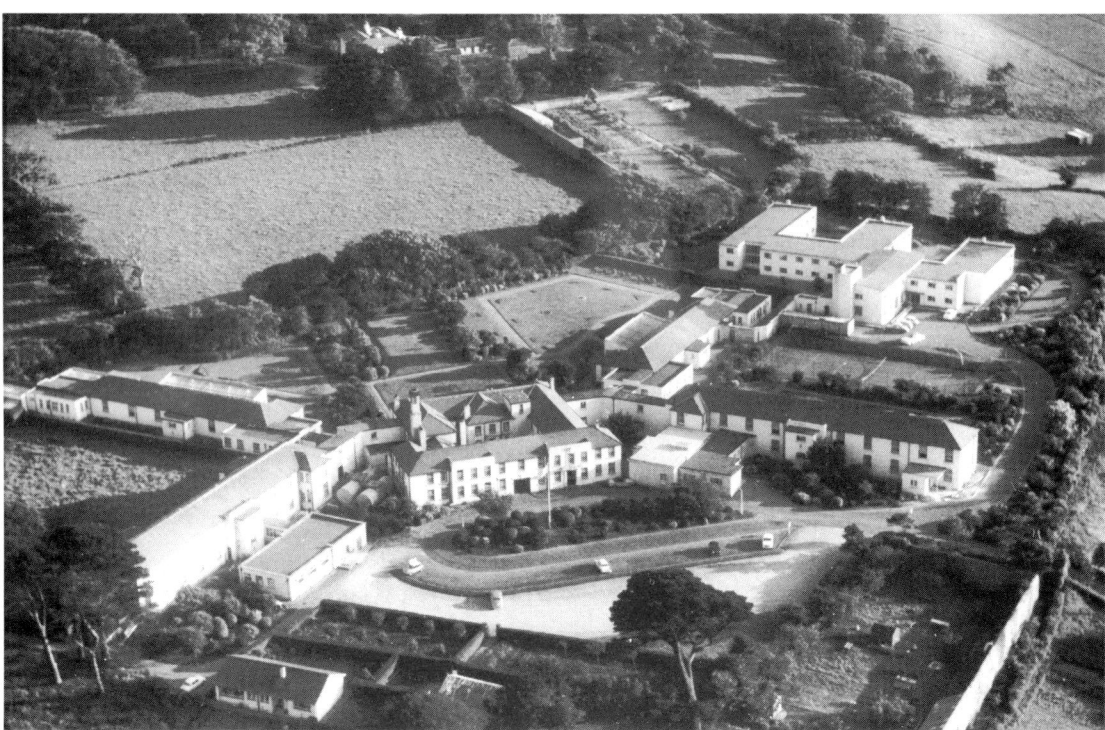

Then and now - the Princess Elizabeth Hospital shortly before its opening in June 1949 and with the "Phase 4" extensions nearing completion in early 1992. When the hospital was first opened, there were only three offices, and parking for around twenty cars. (Chapter Ten)

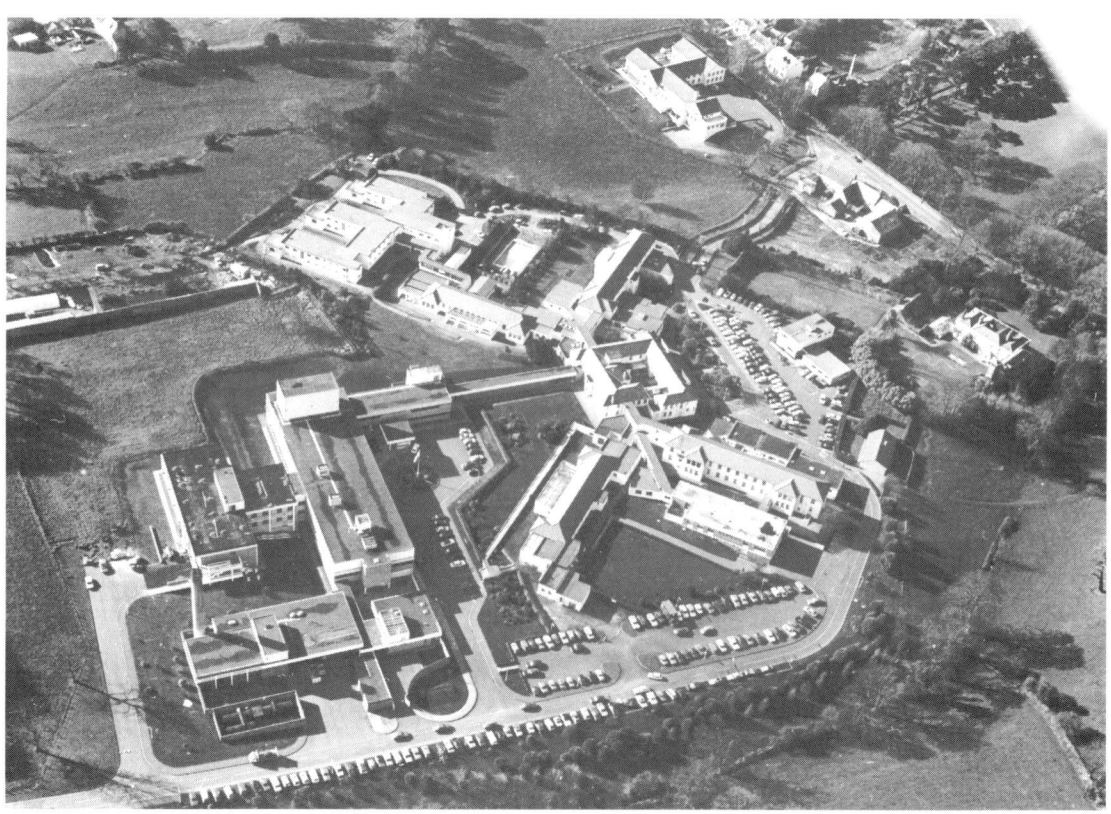

Chapter Sixteen

The Changing Mandate of the Board of Health

Alan Hodgkinson

The evolving role and responsibility of the Board is charted by a series of 'snapshots' of important decisions of the States of Guernsey. In particular the Board's responsibility for managing and developing the islands healthcare institutions and its more recent role in commissioning more comprehensive health services to islanders is examined.

"Starting from here..."

When I came to Guernsey in October 1991, as Chief Executive Officer (Designate) of the Board of Health, I was attracted by the prospect of having the opportunity to use my health management training and experience, in both the public and private sectors, to influence the future provision of health and social services for a whole population.

The system of health care in Guernsey was different from other systems I had experienced. It was primarily a system of private doctors working in public institutions, with a variety a funding and delivery methods, run along local government lines by a political assembly entirely independent of the UK government. It was certainly unique but it appeared to have had no 'master plan' leading to its creation.

In my early years of being Chief Executive I often found myself asking the questions "Why are we in this business?" or "Why is it done this way?" Indeed I still do! One of my favourite expressions, which those who have served on the Board of Health will often have heard me 'quip', is one that I overheard when I was on the Board of the Blackrock Clinic in Dublin:

"Sure, if I was going to go to Dublin, I wouldn't start from here!"

When planning to meet the future health needs of the people of Guernsey we have to start from where we are, not where we would like to be. And so it was for my predecessors (to whom this chapter is dedicated - in gratitude for their achievements). I hope that in years to come my successors will also understand this when criticising my own endeavours.

The role and mandate of the Board of Health has developed incrementally over the past hundred years, in response to the changing health needs of the people of Guernsey and the rapid developments in medicine.

This chapter highlights some of the more important decisions of the States of Deliberation that have added significantly to the responsibilities and authority of the Board, which is now the largest States department.

Diphtheria and disease control

As well chronicled elsewhere in this book, the Board was 'born' in a crisis, on 29th December 1899. Its role was to deal with a diphtheria epidemic. The first Chairman was General H Le Cocq and members were Jurat Ozanne, the Rev. Brock, and Messrs Valpied, Collinette, Dorey, Collas and Foote.

The measures introduced by the Dr Brownlea, Guernsey's first Medical Officer of Health, and his successors, Dr Hoare and then Dr Bishop, proved to be effective in bringing the disease under control. In 1903 the King Edward Sanatorium was opened and by 1904 the worst was over. Dr Bishop and the Board then set about improving the health of the people of Guernsey for more than 30 years. Eventually Dr Bishop's persistence and long service was rewarded in 1934, the year of his retirement, by the introduction of the *'Loi Relative à la Sante Publique'* - for the first time giving legislative force to support the work of the MoH.

Rats and refuse

In February 1935 the States had before them a requete on the question of the destruction of rats. A committee was established for this purpose, which reported back in October of the same year. Two parishes reported that they were unaware of any rat infested areas and four parishes indicated several localities where rats were very prevalent, particularly along douits and waterways. The older parts of St Peter Port were badly infested, especially those areas served by the brick sewers.

They reported " *The rat is a danger to human life,* a *carrier of epidemic diseases, a prolific breeder, of disgusting habits and a destroyer of food and property."*

The Committee recommended that the powers vested in the parish Constables be extended by co-operation with the Board of Health - in view of the concerns for public health. It also recommended the appointment of two men to work for the Board to destroy rats and for the Board to consider the collection and destruction of refuse. The States deferred the decision in favour of further consultation.

Almost two years later, in December 1936, the States debated a joint report from the Board of Health, the Committee for Agriculture and Fisheries and the Destruction of Rats Committee. It was decided to nominate the States Supervisor as an ex-officio member of the Destruction of Rats Committee, and to undertake a survey on the destruction of rats for a one-year period, with the assistance of the MoH. Also, to ask the Royal Court to amend the 1932 Ordinance concerning the *'Destruction of Rats and Mice'* so that the Committee's officers would have the same powers as the parish Constables.

In September 1939, after the outbreak of war, the Committee for the Destruction of Rats reported on the success of its work, with almost 6,000 rats destroyed in 1938. It asked to be made a standing Committee of the States. Unfortunately the work of the States and its Committees was soon to be disrupted by the Occupation.

A new mental hospital

In July 1905, the States had resolved to replace the existing mental asylums (the Town Hospital for men and the Country Hospital for women) with a new building *"in some suitable place in one of the Country Parishes"*. Indeed, in July 1914 the States confirmed their decision to erect such an asylum on the De Putron estate. However, this did not happen (presumably due to the first World War), and the estate was eventually sold for private housing.

The States Asylum Committee resurrected the matter in July 1932, by proposing the appointment of a mental officer for a period of at least one year who would be required to study local conditions and report on the best steps which should be taken.

Dr William Reid McGlashan was duly appointed and he produced a comprehensive report, which was submitted to the States in April 1934. Even for that time it made gruesome reading with its description of the Town Hospital entrance hall as *"...dark and stuffy and one is conscious of an atmosphere of darkness and an odour of dampness immediately on entering the building."*

Apart from a fixed basin used by the Matron there were only two fixed washbasin and two fixed baths to serve the whole hospital. He was sorry to see *"that no adequate means of keeping flies off the faces of weakly and senile invalids had been devised, and none of the dormitories, in the true sense of the word, could be described as suitable for serving as a sick or hospital ward."*

The Country Hospital he described as having *"... the appearance of a prison within a prison. The cold stone corridor flanked by fearsome looking cells chills one to the marrow and a mental invalid might well be forgiven for believing that he was being put in a place of punishment instead of in a home of healing."*

"Both the Mental Hospitals as they stand are badly planned for hospital purposes and...with the best will in the world, neither could be economically remodelled to approach anything like accepted present-day standards."

"A new Mental Hospital capable of serving the whole island, built on a site and on a plan which will allow of easy expansion when necessary, will settle the question of providing complete care and treatment for the mental invalids for of the island, and will remove for ever from Guernsey the anxiety which must trouble and torment the social conditions of every highly civilised and Progressive community."

Various sites were considered including Blanche Pierre Lanes, Beaucamp, Beau Sejour and Le Vauquiedor Estate. The latter was described by the President of the Asylum Committee as *"... delightful and ideally placed... its fine aspect and bracing position, combined with its well sheltered and yet quite beautiful surroundings, render it almost uniquely supreme amongst the numerous places visited and viewed by the Committee, who are considering the question of building a new Mental Hospital for the States of Guernsey Mental Health Services."*

The States agreed to the purchase of Vauquiedor Estate and Farm buildings for the sum of £6,500. Dr McGlashan was rewarded for his efforts by the extension on his appointment for a further year.

Planning of the new hospital commenced. In February 1935 the States adopted a tentative scheme prepared by the States' Engineer and voted the sum of £41,800 to meet the estimated cost, including the cost of the connecting sewer to the Foulon main drain. By March 1937 tenders had been received for the construction of the 'Mental Home'. The Mental Health Services Committee provisionally accepted that of Messrs. Hardars, Ltd., of Jersey in the sum of £56,500.

The disparity in costs was explained by Mr E F Laine, States' Engineer as being due to *"the insufficiency of the sketch plan to provide data for a reliable estimate. Lack of a true conception of the full requirements of such an institution, but mainly as regards the cost thereof. The omission from the estimate of items which are now included in the Bills of Quantities and tenders. The unforeseen rise in the cost of materials since the inception of the proposals (ranging from 5 to 60 per cent)."*

In placing this matter before the States in April 1937 the Bailiff stated: "You *will doubtless be only too ready to embrace this opportunity of voting the extra money, so that the scandal of the present inadequate accommodation which is available for these unfortunate members of society may be rectified."*

"I would rather that every other project should be shelved indefinitely than a building of the Mental Home should be delayed one-day, and I therefore confidently leave this matter in your hands in the sincere hope that you will see your way to pass this extra vote so that the work can be proceeded with at once."

With so powerful a plea the outcome was inevitable and the construction of the new Mental Home at Le Vauquiedor was approved.

A new general hospital

In September and November 1938 the Poor Law Inquiry Committee reported to the States, the outcome of which was agreement to adopt in principle the establishment of a new General Hospital designed to serve the needs of the whole island.

The Committee was empowered to negotiate for the absorption of the Victoria Hospital and the Lady Ozanne Maternity home into the proposed General Hospital scheme. If the Victoria hospital authorities agreed to cede their property to the States, this hospital would be used for maternity purposes.

In addition the Committee was authorised to investigate further the possibility of a contributory scheme.

In view of its new role the mandate of the Committee was changed and its name altered to the Island Hospital Committee.

The following sites were under consideration for the General Hospital:

1. The North field of Beau Sejour
2. Field on the West Side off Ville-au-Roi
3. The property known as les Merriennes, St Martin
4. Saumarez Park, Castel
5. The Country Hospital, Castel
6. Any other site

Following inquiries to the British Hospitals Association, Mr E Stanley Hall M.A., F.R.I.B.A., visited the island, people and produced a report, which resulted in the committee putting forward recommendations to the States in November 1938.

The Committee was about to draw up its final report when the outbreak of war made it necessary to reconsider the project. It reported back to the States in January 1940 *"...the Committee feels that in view of the present circumstances the States will not wish to incur the large expenditure visualised as the possible cost of an island hospital. Secondly, it is now doubtful whether any contractor would be willing to undertake the construction of the hospital in view of the difficulty of obtaining materials and the alteration in the price of such materials which is bound to occur from time to time. It has been suggested that, even if no further steps are taken at present towards the construction of the hospital, inquiry should continue into the possibilities of a contributory scheme for hospital treatment. It is difficult, however, to visualise what the circumstances on the island and its inhabitants will be at the end of the war and what effect the war will have on the running costs of hospital management. As the basis of any contributory scheme must depend on such circumstances, it is felt the consideration of this matter should also be deferred."*

The States agreed that the Committee's mandate should be suspended for the duration of the war and all work ceased. The scheme for building a new general hospital, as had been contemplated, would have cost approximately £200,000.

Preparing for war

Only five days after the declaration of war the Air Raid Precautions Committee reported on the establishment of the 'War Hospital'.

Within 24 hours of the declaration of war, the Country Hospital had been taken over by order of his Excellency the Lieutenant Governor, in the exercise of the powers conferred upon him by the *Emergency War Regulations (Guernsey)*, 1939. The existing patients had been transferred to the Town Hospital and its pauper inmates either billeted out or transferred to the Town Institution.

After a further two days the Country Hospital had been completely reorganised to provide a minimum of 190 beds, with emergency equipment and staffing. The hospital was ready to receive patients on the 8th September 1939 and continued in use throughout and until well after the war, known as the Emergency Hospital.

Reconstitution and Review

The Island was liberated on the 9th May 1945 and five months later the Board of Health was reconstituted by the States and given a much wider mandate:

1. *To deal with all matters relating to the health of the island and Hospital administration therein;*

2. *To embrace the duties previously performed by the Island Hospital Investigation Committee, the Emergency Hospital Board, the existing Board of Health, the Committee for the Collection and Disposal of Refuse, and the Committee for the Destruction of Rats;*

3. *To embrace the duties of the Mental Health Services Board as soon as The Mental Treatment Law (Guernsey) 1939 was amended by Order in Council;*

4. *To confer with the Public Assistance Authority Hospital Board, regarding the transfer of their duties to the Board of Health.*

This was to be the mandate of the Board for more than fifty years.

The Board then comprised seven sitting members of the States and the first President was Dr A N Symons, who had been President in office prior to the Occupation.

On Christmas Eve, 1945 the States, at the request of the Board of Health, agreed to ask the Home Office to send an Advisory Council of Experts to visit the Island to advise on future health and hospital services in Guernsey. This important report was to be pivotal in shaping the future of Guernsey's health and hospital services.

Towards a comprehensive health service

The Advisory Council of three experts (Dr G Bourne, Dr F Grundy and Mr J A Beardsall) visited in February 1946 for one week. The States considered their report in April 1946. The report envisaged the complete unification and integration of health and medical services. It identified the following bed need for Guernsey's envisaged post-war population of up to 40,000:

Acute Hospital Beds	140
Chronic Sick	50
Infectious Diseases	20
Tuberculosis	28
Maternity	33
Mental Diseases	70-80

The report also classified three specialist medical services needed for the Island's population:

1. Off-island centres London Teaching Hospitals where patients could be treated for rarer conditions: the cost of transport to be met by the States and the cost of treatment to be *'worked out to fit in with the future health services of England.'*

2. Regular visits by specialists from London Teaching Hospitals in the disciplines of General Medicine, General Surgery, Orthopaedic Surgery, and Gynaecology and Obstetrics. Travel and accommodation costs to be met by the States plus a fee for attending. A Consulting Pathologist to whom particular specimens would be sent for investigation was also envisaged.

3. The development of the General Practitioner specialists to organise themselves in teams to cover surgery, paediatrics, obstetrics and possibly clinical pathology and ophthalmology.

The report recommended the introduction of a comprehensive scheme designed to make financial provision during ill health. This would enable patients to have a free choice of doctor. Reciprocal arrangements with the new scheme to be devised for England and Wales were recommended.

The main recommendations of the report centred on the provision of a modern and efficient General Hospital, which it was recommended, should be situated at Le Vauquiedor Hospital - instead of this being used for the mentally ill.

The General Hospital required a modern operating theatre, diagnostic X-ray Department, laundry and staff quarters to be added plus a private block *'in order that the private and routine hospital work of the staff shall be done at the same centre.'* The authors even suggested a name for the new general hospital. *'Was not St. Sampson the Island's patron saint:?'*

Staffing of the new general hospital was also considered in the report, which recommended:

1. A resident medical officer with surgical experience
2. A full time physiotherapist (with no private practice)
3. Pensions for nurses
4. A nurse training school
5. An Almoner (medical social worker)
6. A full time laboratory technician (for the Public Health Lab.)
7. A trained caterer
8. A chief executive officer or 'House Governor and Secretary'

It was recommended that the Victoria Hospital become the maternity unit, with a resident obstetric officer to replace the responsibilities of GPs. A visiting psychiatrist was recommended for the mental health services. Additional staff was also recommended to support the MoH including a deputy, a dental officer and two health visitors.

Finally the report concluded by noting that Guernsey had no body to supervise and regulate the medical profession and recommended that the States make application to the Privy Council for an extension of the jurisdiction of the General Medical Council to include the medical affairs of the Island.

An appendix to the report contained a summary of the conditions observed by the visitors when inspecting the island's hospitals. Today it makes grim reading - an example is the description of the operating theatre at the Emergency Hospital:

> *The present theatre arrangements are unsuitable and need extensive remodelling, for the following reasons:*
>
> 1. *There is no separate sterilising room. The present arrangements for sterilising dressings are unsuitable.*
> 2. *There are no scrubbing up and sluice room facilities.*
> 3. *There is no special anaesthetic room.*
> 4. *There are no nurses' changing rooms. The present structure does not lend itself to asepsis.*

New hospitals planned

The island clearly needed a new General Hospital. So in April 1946 the States agreed to the appointment of a consultant hospital architect, to advise on the practicability and estimated cost of converting the Vauquiedor Mental Hospital into a General Hospital and the Emergency Hospital into a Mental Hospital. Alternatively, converting the Emergency Hospital to the requirements of a modern hospital and turning the Children's Home into a nurses' home, or building of a new nurses' home. The architect was also to advise on converting the Victoria Hospital to a Maternity Home.

Mr S W Milburn, F.R.I.B.A. visited the island from June 4th to June 8th 1946 and inspected the following institutions:

> Le Vauquiedor Hospital.
> The Emergency Hospital
> Men's Mental Wards
> The Children's Home
> King Edward Sanatorium
> Victoria Hospital
> Military Hospital at Ville-au-Roi

He subsequently reported to the Board of Health and his *"Report upon the proposed re-organisation of the Hospital Services"* was attached to the Billet D'Etat considered by the States on 11th December 1946. He confined his report *"to the larger and more essential issues under consideration"* which, in summary, were as follows:

1. Converting the Vauquiedor Hospital into a General Hospital

"This hospital, a modern building, lends itself well to a comparatively economical conversion into a first-class General Hospital. The essentials of a modern General Hospital are all there, centralised services, a sunny exposure for the patients wards, well arranged ward units and Northern entrances for Patients, Staff and Goods."

He recommended the provision of a bed and service lift; a sluice room in each ward; an operating theatre; X-ray department; mortuary; private ward; the provision of a separate nurses' and maids' homes; a nurse Training school and space for car parking. The scheme would provide accommodation for 124 acute and 20 private patients plus 90 nurses and maids. The total cost was estimated at £106,000.

2. Converting the Emergency Hospital into a Mental Hospital

"No special difficulties present themselves in converting this building into a modern mental hospital to provide accommodation for 80 mental patients of both sexes. The buildings are old but being originally designed in the workhouse or public institution type of plan, easily adapt themselves to accommodate the chronic type of patient who can be up and about most of the day."

He proposed nursing staff accommodation on the top floor; a passenger lift; chronic male and female wards on the first floor; acute male patients in the reconstructed "Asylum" block and acute female patients in the reconstruction of the ground floor of the children's wing. The total cost of this conversion was estimated at £40,600.

3. The Building of an Island Hospital Laundry

"The centralising of all Hospital Laundry Services in one building would undoubtedly prove a measure of some considerable economy and efficiency, and I have given this matter very careful consideration. The site I suggest should be the low land North-West of the Vauquiedor Hospital... Accommodation would be provided to wash for the whole of the patients and staff..."

The design of the central laundry was to include separate wash-houses for general, foul, and infected linen as well as a separate area for staff garments. The estimated cost of the scheme, including buildings, steams supply and machinery was £43,000.

4. Improvement of Present Laundry at the Emergency Hospital

Adaptations costing approximately £2,600 were proposed so that *"this laundry can continue to deal with the Island's hospital requirements for a number of years."*

5. Converting the Emergency Hospital into a General Hospital

" ... is not a proposition capable of a satisfactory solution. The children's home could be converted to provide staff accommodation, but I think it would be a pity to disturb the working of this very happy, well-arranged institution."

6. Converting the Victoria to Hospital into Maternity Home
"This is a fine building and was comparatively small alterations will convert quite easily into a modern antenatal clinic and maternity nursing home. " It was recommended that the hand-operated lift be electrified.

7. King Edward Sanatorium
"... eminently suited for its purpose."

8. Immediate Policy
"Conditions are such as the emergency hospital, especially in regard to the important provision for operating, General Nursing and food storage, that they should not be allowed to continue for a minute longer than necessary.

During the course of my professional studies, I have either visited or have obtained detailed knowledge of the majority of English and Continental and American General Hospitals, and in no case are medical, nursing and administrative staffs called upon to work under such difficult conditions.

In the policy letter the President of the Board of Health wrote:

"To provide a new hospital, three alternatives would appear possible.
  1. *An entirely new building*
  2. *Reconstructing the present Emergency Hospital*
  3. *Adapting the Vauquiedor to a General Hospital and the present Emergency Hospital to a Mental Hospital"*

"It is not to be believed that the States, when they have realised the poor conditions under which the sick of the island have to be attended, would desire to prolong the position further.

The withholding of the Vauquiedor buildings from the mental patients is the only strong argument against this Scheme. It is, however, necessary to strike a balance between the mental cases, who are limited in number, and the many cases who month by month will pass in and come through the General Hospital. At the emergency hospital some 1,500 patients have been admitted each year."

11th December 1946 was a momentous day for the Board of Health. The equivalent of its first 'site development plan' had been approved. In total the States voted £113,000 for the conversion of the Vauquiedor Hospital to a General Hospital, including the purchase of X-ray apparatus and furniture.

The Board also received £40,600 for the conversion of the Emergency Hospital buildings for use as a Mental Hospital, to house 80 patients of both sexes, plus £2,600 to upgrade the hospital's existing laundry.

A further £15,107 was voted for the purchase of the Victoria Hospital, its upgrading and furnishing for use as the Island Maternity Home.

In May 1948 the Board of Health reported to the States that work was proceeding on the hospital at Le Vauquiedor and it would be ready to open as are the island's General Hospital towards the end of 1948. The States agreed, subject to the consent of her Royal Highness the Princess Elizabeth, that the hospital should be named after her.

The transfer of patients from the Emergency Hospital to the Princess Elizabeth Hospital took place on November 27th, 1948.

The refurbishment of the Victoria Hospital proved to be much more costly than anticipated and the Board of Health had to report to the States in March 1949 that the project was heavily overspent. Moreover, it was anticipated that even when converted it would still be inadequate to meet the needs of the island. Thus the Board considered it would need to come forward with plans to extend or replace the Maternity Unit before it had opened!

The maternity section remained at the Emergency Hospital until the new maternity unit at Amherst was ready to receive them on October 7th, 1949.

The Board of Health returned to the States in January 1950 and obtained approval to convert the Emergency Hospital to a Mental Hospital with 100 beds and to upgrade the hospital's laundry by the installation of a new boiler and washing machine.

Thus it was that the hospital at Le Vauquiedor became The Princess Elizabeth Hospital, and not the mental hospital originally planned for that site.

Reciprocal Health Agreement

Although patients sent to England for hospital treatment had been receiving such treatment without any charge since the commencement of the NHS on 5th July 1948, it was not until May 1950 that the Board reported to the States on *'Proposed reciprocal arrangements for hospital and medical treatment, etc. with the United Kingdom.'*

Agreement had been reached between the Board and the island doctors whereby the Board would undertake, on specific terms, to meet the medical charges incurred by doctors in the treatment of bona fide visitors to the island from England, Wales, Scotland, Northern Ireland and the Isle of Man. In addition hospital treatment would be given and X-ray facilities be at the disposal of the doctors where necessary without charge to the visitor-patient. Dental and specialised ophthalmic treatment would be excluded from this arrangement.

In return the United Kingdom had agreed to pay for Channel Islanders being treated in NHS hospitals in the South West Region (except those which related to mental health and mental deficiency, for which payment would have to be made by the States of Guernsey) whenever adequate hospital facilities did not exist in the Channel Islands. Channel Island residents were to be afforded equal priority for admission as if they were UK residents. The costs of the boat fares to and from the islands were to be paid by the patients.

The agreement with the local doctors was to be reviewed at the end of 1951. It was difficult to estimate what the annual cost of this agreement with the local doctors would be to the Board. Doctors would be reimbursed five shillings for surgery appointment or seven shillings and sixpence for a home visit. It had been agreed however that a total ceiling of £8,000 per annum would apply.

The States agreed that the new arrangements should come into force on the 1st June 1950 and to vote the State's Board of Health the credit of £8,000 to cover the cost of treatment of visitors to the island for that year.

This historic agreement, which has now been in operation for almost 50 years, has meant that thousands of Channel Islanders have received 'free' treatment in the United Kingdom, the cost of such treatment effectively being met by the respective Channel Island Health Authorities by a 'balancing' mechanism of meeting the costs of treating visitors to the islands.

Its introduction in Guernsey at that time seems, to the author of this article, somewhat inequitable. It meant that UK visitors could receive 'free' treatment by the island's general practitioners whereas local residents had to pay. Also, a local resident could receive free treatment in the United Kingdom hospitals whereas if they remained in Guernsey they would have to pay their doctor's fees. This anomalous situation was not to be rectified until the 1990s, by the introduction of the compulsory specialist health insurance scheme, followed later by the reintroduction of GP charges to UK visitors.

'Strike' by Princess Elizabeth Hospital nurses

An emergency meeting of the Board took place at 4pm on 9th July 1957, following the receipt of a petition, signed by 21 nurses and a member of the Pathology Department staff, by Miss M H Dann the Acting Matron.

The petition stated: *" The above nurses refuse to enter the Dining Room as from tomorrow 10.7.57. until a matter is called to discuss the food problem"*. A copy had been forwarded to the local newspapers in advance and an article had been published.

There had been complaints about 'salty' tongue, streaky bacon, canned tomatoes and other concerns for quite some time. The Board had been investigating the matter for several weeks and even sampling meals themselves. However, it appeared that three ward sisters had been aware of the petition and that it had been handed to the media and the Board found this to be *'disgraceful and unprofessional'*.

The Board interviewed some of the petitioners, then a message was received that the other staff concerned had requested a mass meeting with the Board. The Board adjourned to the Dining room to meet them. The staff said they had not been informed of the Board's investigations into the poor food. This was put down to poor communications.

The Members returned to the Boardroom and were still primarily concerned with the breach of discipline. They decided to dismiss the staff nurse who was spokesperson of the group, having *'lost confidence'* in her and to report the ward sisters to the Royal College of Nursing for a *'lack of responsibility'*.

The Board met again on 11th July to consider a letter from 12 nurses who were threatening resignation unless their colleague was reinstated. It met with the staff concerned the same afternoon. The staff were told that the Board would not reinstate their colleague. Their resignations were accepted immediately and they were asked to vacate the nurses' home as soon as possible.

The next day the Board reconvened to be told that the dockers were threatening to go on strike in sympathy with the dismissed nurses. They agreed to the setting up of an independent tribunal by the Bailiff *'to enquire and report on the dismissal and resignations at the Princess Elizabeth Hospital in connection with the food strike'*.

The results of the Enquiry were reported to the Board on 28th July and it was not good news. The Enquiry felt that the Board should have averted the situation that led to the Enquiry. Having agreed to the setting up of the Enquiry there was little choice for the Members but to consider tendering their resignations at the next States meeting. They decided to sleep on it overnight.

Next day the Board met again to decide what action they should take. They decided to do the honourable thing. A statement was prepared for the President to read out at the next States meeting.

On the morning of the 30th July the dismissed Staff Nurse and her resigned colleagues met with the Assistant Matron and apologised to her. All seemed anxious to put the events of the past weeks behind them and pledged their loyalty to the Hospital if they were reinstated. The Board was informed of this at its meeting that afternoon and agreed not to accept the notice of resignation from the 12 nurses and to reinstate the Staff Nurse.

The Board's President sent the following letter to the Bailiff:

> *'The Board has now considered most carefully the report of the Committee set up by the Bailiff on July 12th to enquire into certain matters concerning The Princess Elizabeth Hospital and we have unanimously come to the conclusion that our duty plainly lies in the submission of our resignation to the States. This we now do.*
>
> *We have the honour to request, therefore, that you will be so good as to lay this matter before the States at your early convenience. Please accept our assurance that in so resigning we have no desire to cause any kind of inconvenience or embarrassment to anyone and we are prepared to continue in office until the States have had a reasonable opportunity to elect a new Board.'*

The States considered the letter at their meeting of 18th September 1957 and decided **not** to accept the resignations. So the Board survived but one feels that a salutary lesson must have been learned by all parties on the importance of good industrial relations in health services.

Extensions to the Princess Elizabeth Hospital

In December 1983 the States accepted in principle the Board of Health's plan for health care to meet the needs of the Bailiwick of Guernsey over the next 10 years. On 25th October 1985 the States approved in principle the Board's proposals for extensions to the Princess Elizabeth Hospital.

Phase 3A (workshops and engineering stores) was completed in 1987 and in May of that year the States agreed to re-phase the remainder of the works as follows:

>   Phase 3B (link block to original hospital)
>   Phase 3C (Laundry)
>   Phase 4 (Main hospital extension)

In April 1989 the Board of Health requested the States to authorise them to utilise Higgs and Hill Management Contracting Limited as the management contractors for phase 4 of the Princess Elizabeth hospital extensions. The States agreed and work on phase 4 commenced. It was to provide:

>   Accident & Emergency Department
>   Radiology Department
>   Children's Ward
>   Maternity Ward
>   Private and Isolation Beds
>   Central Kitchen and Dining Room

The main arguments in favour of the new facilities were that the existing departments were outdated and not coping with the workload. There was also a 'prophetic' statement about the anticipated difficulty in recruiting staff to work in health services.

> *"Alongside Guernsey's own recruitment problems, there is the international problem of the reduced number of young people leaving school to start work and care for the increasingly large number of older people, who are major users of health and social services.*
>
> *As we enter the 21st century there will be a steady growth in number of people over the age of 65 - and particularly an increase in the number of people over the age of 75 who are greater users of health care resources. Against this, the lower birth rate means that there will be a smaller working population to look after the sick and the elderly.*
>
> *Health services have in the past traditionally been staffed primarily by women: the large range of careers now open to women has led to a very considerable reduction in number going into nursing and allied health care professions.*

Despite initiatives to improve recruitment and retention of staff, the Board still needs to reorganise its services so that in the future they can be maintained with the minimum number of staff: at present rather the number of sites makes duplication of staff unavoidable."

In December 1989 Board of Health reported to the States on the estimated cost of extensions to the Princess Elizabeth Hospital and also requested the States agreement to the building of a new laundry on the Princess Elizabeth Hospital site. The estimated costs were as follows:

| Phase 4 | £17,769,479 |
| Laundry | £ 2,278,499 |

The States agreed to the projects and allocated the funds to the Board.

Phase 4 was completed early in 1992 and was formally opened by HRH The Duchess of Gloucester, after whom the dining room is named.

Financial and staffing problems

In November 1989 the Board of Health reported to the States on order to give an update on progress made on its 1983 plan for health care. It also took the opportunity to recommend to the States the way in which the Board of Health considered health care should be provided in Guernsey in the future and how this should be funded.

The Board reported good progress with centralising on the Princess Elizabeth Hospital site and with increasing the number of beds at the Duchess of Kent House - from 48 to 100, in 1986. The Board had hoped that it would be possible to release the Castel Hospital for other purposes but this had not been possible. Considerable progress had been made in developing community service for the elderly and the mentally ill. The health promotion unit had been established in 1988 and the Board had taken on responsibility for the school medical service and school dental service in 1989.

The report showed that between 1982 and 1988 the Board of Health's total expenditure had increased by 87 per cent (34 per cent when adjusted for inflation). The majority of this increase was in staff salaries. The continuing rise in expenditure was of great concern to the Board as demonstrated in the following quotation:

> *"... the Board of Health fully accepts that expenditure cannot be permitted to continue increasing at this level and in an uncontrolled way, as the time will come when the amount of money provided by the States for health care has to be reduced - either because of the level of States' income has reduced or because the money is more urgently required for other purposes."*

> *"Guernsey is fortunate in the availability of good standard health care but if the services are to be maintained and extended in line with the development of new technology then the States has to face the fact that it is impossible to contain costs. Although the patient pays the doctor a fee this is for his professional advice and time. The treatment which he prescribes will be funded either through the Pharmaceutical Scheme (if it is a drug for treatment outside Hospital) or through the Board of Health, which totally meet the cost of all drugs, treatment, medical supplies, investigations, and services provided in the acute hospital services. If, for example, the doctor recommends blood tests, X-rays and subsequently in-patient treatment, all this is funded by the States. The Board of Health does not have control of the doctor's clinical decisions."*

> *"In the National Health Service, when the money runs out the service stops and beds are closed. Members of the states will be familiar with many reports in the UK national press of patients, including children, who have been denied the treatment they urgently need, sometimes with fatal consequences.*

> *The Board does not feel that county's services should be run in this way. It is not prepared to take this drastic step on to deny patients treatment without the prior knowledge and support of the States, so that people are aware of the reasons and in the knowledge that the States will share responsibility for the outcome. Alternatively, a system must be found which permit patients to receive the treatment they require but which does not produce an unrestricted demand on stage resources."*

With regards to staffing the Board's report stated:

> *"...the immediate crisis facing the service is a shortage of staff and the difficulty of maintaining services. Guernsey now has full employment, and there are many alternatives well-paid and attractive post available to those who have traditionally worked in the health services. Similar difficulties for trained staff are being experienced by health authorities in the south England, but they have the advantage of being able to recruit any skilled workers from immigrant communities where unemployment still exists.*

> *In Guernsey the Board is facing a shortage of unskilled manual staff as well as a shortage of skilled and professionally qualified staff. It is unable to recruit staff within the Island and because of the wish of the States to control population, it is limited in the number of staff it is able to bring in from the UK..."*

When considering the future funding of a health services the Board was of the view that the acute hospital should be run on the lines of a private hospital, with charges being introduced to finance the services provided. It suggested that the State's Insurance Authority *'should be requested to report to the States as soon as possible with the details and cost of suitable health insurance schemes, which would include cover for charges macle for acute hospital services.'*

The debate of this report fashioned the direction of future health services in Guernsey by passing the following resolutions:

> 1. That the residents of Guernsey and Alderney shall continue to have access to health care services without the imposition by the States of arbitrary financial or other constraints until such time as the Board of Health have determined and the state have approved charges for hospital services.
>
> 2. To request the State's Insurance Authority to report to the States as soon as the States have accepted the proposals of the Board of Health for the introduction of charges for acute services with details and costs of suitable health insurance schemes which would include cover for charges made for acute hospital services.

The scene was set for the introduction of a health insurance scheme for Guernsey residents.

Health Insurance Scheme

The Board of Health and the Social Insurance Authority both reported to the States on the 29th April 1992. The Board of Health proposed *'that charges be introduced for all acute services provided by the State Board of Health including charges for in-patient nights, day patient attendances, maternity care, out-patient treatments, use of operating theatres, radiological examinations, pathology tests and surgical implants which will become the property of the patient, provided that these charges could be recovered from a Health Insurance Scheme.'*

The Social Insurance Authority reported on its proposals for the introduction of an Island-wide compulsory health insurance scheme that was to cover medical costs and hospital charges for residents who had lived in Guernsey and Alderney for 26 weeks in aggregate at any time. It was proposed that the insurance cover would be provided by Norwich Union Healthcare Ltd and the estimated cost of the scheme in 1993 was £28 million per annum.

After a very long debate the States made the interesting decision of accepting the Board of Health's proposals to introduce acute hospital charges but only agreeing the Social Insurance Authority's proposals in principle - directing them to report back to the States within 12 months with new recommendations *"taking full account of the various issues raised during the debate on this article"*.

The President of the Social Security Authority (previously Social Insurance Authority) made a statement at the state's meeting of 31st March 1993 in which he gave notice that the authority would be unable to report back within 12 months as directed *'owing to the many issues which the Authority had to address to accord with the state's resolution.'*

The Authority finally reported to the States in January 1994 then setting out options for the way forward including the extent of insurance cover, the insurer and the method of funding. The authority had a preferred option, which was for a scheme to cover specialist medical care fees only, administered by the Social Security Authority itself. The Authority and the Board of Health would negotiate pre-payment contracts with the Medical Specialists Group and other providers of specialist medical services. The scheme would be funded by an earnings based system for persons in employment, including a contribution from employers, and an income based system for persons not in employment, including persons of 65 and over.

The maximum additional contribution to be paid in 1995 was estimated to be in the region of £4.14 per week and this was to provide funds to purchase specialist medical services, estimated to cost £5M p.a.

The Board of Health supported the Authority's new proposals since it saw advantage in extending its role as a purchaser of health care services. It envisaged that the Board would be able to choose between providing services itself, contracting with others to provide them on island, or indeed contracting with providers to provide them off island, including Jersey and the UK.

The States liked the new proposals, which they agreed in principle. The Authority was asked to report back as soon as possible with detailed proposals and the decision to introduce charges for acute hospital services was rescinded.

The Authority reported back to the States in June 1995 with detailed proposals for a health insurance scheme to cover all residents of Guernsey and Alderney against the cost of specialist medical care. It was proposed to enter into a contract for seven years duration with the Medical Specialist Group at cost fixed in real terms at £4.73M p.a.

The States liked the new proposals, which were approved. In addition the States agreed to additional staff and associated costs required by the Board of Health for the anticipated increase in workload at the Princess Elizabeth Hospital.

The compulsory Specialist Health Insurance scheme was introduced on 1st January 1996. As predicted the workload of the Princess Elizabeth Hospital grew in the first year by 13 per cent and in the second year of the scheme by a further 7 per cent. This 'surge' in workload was felt to be due to the fact that people could now access secondary medical care, without the fear of the bill from the specialist. Equity of access to acute hospital treatment had finally been achieved in Guernsey. It was now 'free at the point of delivery' only 48 years after the creation of the NHS in the UK.

A New Mandate

In 1997 the States agreed a new mandate for the Board of Health as follows:

'1. To advise the States on matters relating to:

- *health education,*

- *promoting, protecting and improving environmental and public health;*

- *preventing or diagnosing and treating illness, disease and disability;*

- *caring for the sick, old, infirm and those with disabilities.*

2. *To develop, present to the States for approval and to implement other policies on the above matters for the provision of services, introduction of legislation and other appropriate measures which contribute to the achievement of strategic and corporate objectives.*

3. *To exercise powers and duties conferred on it by extant legislation and States resolutions.*

4. *To be accountable to the States for the management and safeguarding of public funds and other resources entrusted to it'.*

This mandate makes much clearer the wide role and specific responsibilities of the Board of Health not just *'all matters relating to the health of the island and Hospital administration therein'* as laid down in the previous mandate.

Still "...going to Dublin"

So, what next for the Board of Health? Well, referring to my regular 'quip', despite starting from here, we are still intent on 'going to Dublin'.

In July 1999 the Board asked the States of Guernsey to approve its new Site Development Plan, which it did. The purpose of the plan is *'to enable the Board to provide modern services of an appropriate standard to meet the health care needs of the population and to attract the best staff to deliver the services which should be provided locally.'*

The outcome of implementing the plan will be that all acute hospital services will be located in suitable accommodation on the Princess Elizabeth Hospital site, together with the base for community children's services and community nursing; this will vacate Lukis House and the Castel Hospital. All patient areas for older people will be on the ground floor and the need for staff residential accommodation and training facilities will also be met.

The total cost of the plan is £30M and it will take at least seven years to achieve. By the end of that period all of the Board services should be provided in suitable buildings - something that it has clearly never been able to do before.

What of the future? With an ageing population demand for health services will continue to grow. A declining workforce will mean that recruitment and retention of staff will be a continuing difficulty. Expectations of the public will continue to rise as new cures and treatments are discovered and developed. New drugs and treatment modalities will be costly. The way that healthcare is funded and provided will constantly be changing in an effort to improve efficiency and effectiveness without adversely affecting access or equity. The Board will hold a central position on all of these issues as purchaser, provider, employer and legislator. It will continue to affect the quality of the lives of the citizens of Guernsey hopefully for the better.

Within the confines of this chapter it has not been possible to highlight all of the achievements of the Board of Health over the past 100 years. A few significant changes, together with a few interesting anecdotes are all that space would permit.

One thing seems certain, however, without the Board of Health and its ability to influence the States of Deliberation, the people of Guernsey would not enjoy the range and quality of health care services that they have available to them today. In particular they would not have their hospitals and community services, the health insurance scheme, joint surgery, breast screening, abortion, food fit for consumption, a reduction in smoking, cleaner air and less pollution, fewer rats and no diphtheria!

I have been privileged to play a small part in the development of health services in Guernsey over the past years and have enjoyed writing this chapter. Learning about the past has helped me to better understand our starting point and how we got here.

Now, does anyone know a better way of getting to Dublin?

Appendix Presidents of the Board of Health

States Board of Health: Constituted 1899

Date	President	
1900	General Hubert Le Cocq	
1901	W. Mansell MacCulloch	
1902	John N. Brouard	(Acting President)
1902-1913	John N. Brouard	
1914	G.E. Kinnersly	
1915	G.H. Le Mottée	(Acting President)
1916-1921	G.H. Le Mottée	(President, Comite pour la Sanitation)
1922-1927	G.E. Kinnersly	(President, Comite pour la Sanitation)
1928	Arthur Dorey	
1929	P.S. Mesny	(Acting President)
1930-1931	Arthur Dorey	
1932	P.S. Mesny	(Acting President)
1933	Arthur Dorey	
1934	P.S. Mesny	(Acting President)
1935-1937	Arthur Dorey	
1939	Dr A.N. Symons	

The Board of Health was reconstituted in 1945 under the Presidency of Dr A.N. Symons, the President in Office before the Occupation.

1945-1948	Dr A.N. Symons	
1949-1952	H.G. Stevenson	
1952-1958	Colin J. McCathie	
1958-1960	H.R. Bichard	
1960	A.F.S. Mackay	(Acting President)
1961-1976	Allan N. Grut	(to 30.04.1976)
1976-1990	J.R.R. Henry	
1991-1994	R.M. Chilcott	(from 30.01.1991 to 04.1994)
1994-1998	Mrs S.M. Plant	(from 05.1994)
1998	Brian Russell	

Medical Officers of Health

1899-1900	Dr John Brownlea
1900-1902	Dr E Stanley Hoare
1903-1935	Dr Henry Draper Bishop
1936-1956	Dr Rowan Revell
1957-1960	Dr F Lynch
1961-1967	Dr A Thomas
1968-1981	Dr Geoffrey White
1982-1990	Dr Peter Lawrence
1994	Dr David Jeffs

Board Secretaries, Administrators, Chief Executive Officers

In 1945 it was agreed to request the Board of Administration to appoint an independent Secretary to the Board of Health. Although this post may have been filled before, the first named Secretary on the minutes was Mr H.W. Cochrane in 1950.

1950-1959	H.W. Cochrane	
1960-1974	J.W. Sarre	(to 31.03.1974)
1974-1981	V.E. Luff	(from 01.04.1974)
1982-1992	Mrs Jo Williams	
1992	Mr Alan Hodgkinson	

INDEX

Adulteration of foods 10
Air Charter 154
Air Raid 89, 146
  Precautions 87, 169
Alderney 155
  The Alderney (Application of Legislation) Law 1948 156
  States of 159
Alexandra House 117, 120
Ambulance/s 35, 88, 97
  contribution scheme 145
  motorised 143
  service 92
Amherst 45, 47, 51, 103, 175
Annual Picnic 35, 43
Asthma 140
Aurigny Wing 159
Austin Mr George 26, 27
Auxiliary Fire Service 88

Bairds Mr Mike 28
Ball Mr John 27
Baths 10, 137
BCG Vaccine 72
Black Report 77, 107, 114,
Blanchford Mr Reg 93, 144, 149
Blood donor register 147
Board of Health 7, 39, 77, 84, 93, 102, 113, 121, 157, 160
Bound Dr Harry 140
Breastfeeding 13
Breeches-buoy 148
Brownlea Dr John 3, 6, 166
Bulstrode Dr John 104

Carey Nicholas 51
Central Council (of GDNA) 83, 84
Charter Aircraft 147, 154
Chilcott Conseiller Bob 114, 117
Children's Home 41
Child Guidance Clinic 76
Christmas 36, 37, 44
Cliff Rescue 154
Community Nurses 79, 86
Complementary medicine 140, 142
Consultant Community Paediatrician 77
Contracts
  Renegotiation of 133

Control of Environment Pollution Law 29
Controlling Committee 37, 89, 91, 102
Cost concerns 126

Defibrillators 151
Dene Mr Michael 151
Diamond Jubilee 1, 35
Diphtheria 6, 24, 35, 69, 71, 94, 101, 137
District Nursing Association 71, 79, 81
Douzaines 11
  opposition of 7
Draper Bishop Dr Henry 8, 16, 25, 70, 135
Dunkirk 89

"Eight Pound Grant" 127
Emergency Hospital 59, 88, 91, 102, 169
Environmental health officers 28, 29
Evacuation 89, 146, 156
Eye examinations 73

Fear of War 87
First aid room 150
First World War 15, 33, 52
Floraville 46, 63
Flying Christine 147, 148, 153
Food legislation 27

General Nursing Council 80
German instruments 156
Gibson Dr Dick 102
Global environment 28
Grande Maison Road surgery 116
Group practice 99, 112
Grow Limited 67
Guerin Collection 3
Guernsey Council on Alcoholism 61
Guernsey Healing Fellowship 140
Guernsey Social Security Authority (GSSA) (formerly SIA) 130, 181

Hayward Foundation 148
Health
  Centre concept 157
  statistics 9
  visitors 13, 72, 85
Herve Mr Ronald 150
Hoare Dr E Stanley 8
Holistic care 141
Home confinements 155

Hospital
  Abolition of charges 125
  Castel 104, 138
  Country 57, 91, 119, 167
  Guernsey Cottage 47, 48
  Mignot Memorial 156, 158, 163
  Princess Elizabeth 60, 96, 103, 119, 164, 175, (extension to) 178
  Town 31, 32, 57, 97, 146
  Vauquiedor 103, 109, 171
  Victoria 91, 103, 174
Housing 10

Illegitimate births 137
Immunisation 15, 77
Impey Mr F L 157
Infant mortality rate 4, 10, 12
Infanticide 137
Infectious diseases 15
Influenza epidemic 14
Inshore rescue boat 148
Inspectors of Nuisances 23
"Island medical law" 136

Jubilee Home 157

Knackery 25, 139

Lady Ozanne Maternity Home 53, 54, 91, 103
Le Cocq General H 3, 8, 166
Legislation 11
Les Cotils Christian Centre 142
Liberation 72
Life expectancy 3
Loi Relative à la Sante Publique 12, 26, 29, 166
Loi Relative a la l'Instruction Primaire 70
Long-term care 132
Lunatic Asylum 32, 41
Lung cancer rate 17

Maternal deaths 13
Maternity care 92
McGlashan Dr William 59, 70, 103
Measles 69
Meat Inspectors 139
Medical Expenses Assistance Scheme (MEAS) 127, 133
Medical Officer of Health 6, 23, 58, 91, 136
  Deputy 157
Medical Specialist Group 78, 99, 124
Medical Staff Committee 107, 116

Mental Deficiency Committee 63
Mental Health
  Committee 103
  Week 60
Midwives 14, 82
Mignot Rev. Peter 155
Mignot Centre 67
Milk 13, 21, 75, 137
  in schools scheme 71, 75
Milnes Walker Report 105
Mobile radar unit 149, 153
Mothers Clinic 13
Munich crisis 87

National Health Service 99, 111, 180
'New mandate' 182
Night baking 26, 28
1959 Scheme 123
1991 Census 133
Norwich Union Scheme 129, 130
NSPCC 76
Nuffield Trust 157
Nurse training school 171
Nurses strike 176

Occupation 26, 36, 71, 156, 166
Ordinance Provisional a la Sante Publique 26
Ordonnance ayant rapport aux Sages Femmes 82
Opthalmic Group 131
Orthoptic treatment 73

Paramedic skills 151, 152
Pathology 105
Pharmaceutical service 123
Physiotherapy 132
Poor Law Board 31, 34, 143
Primary Care Committee 115, 117
Prescription charges 125
Prince of Wales 140
Princess Elizabeth 109, 110
Psychology Services 61
Public Health
  Act 1848 23
  Act 1875 12, 24, 26
Punishments 36, 59

Queen Elizabeth II 158
Queen Elizabeth the Queen Mother 106, 110
Queens Institute 81

Radiology 104
Radios (two way) 147

Rationing 95
Rats 166
  Destruction of Rats Committee 166
Reciprocal Agreement 107, 175
Recompression chamber 148
Recruitment problems 62, 178
Registration
  of Cause of Death 9
  of nurses 80
Reports
  Black 77, 107, 114
  Peat Marwick Mitchell (PMM) 126
  Thompson 61
Revell Dr Rowan 16, 26, 71, 93
Robinson Dr E Laurie 47, 54
Royal Guernsey Militia 1
Royal Court 6, 25, 102

Salisbury Dr Barbara 60, 74
Sanatorium King Edward 8, 15, 58, 122, 136, 144, 174
Sanitary reform 23
Sanitary Inspector 25
Sark 93
School
  Dental Service 72, 74
  Medical Officer 70
  Medical Services 77
School nurse 70, 71, 73, 85
'Screwtape Letters' 142
Sedan Chair 22, 35
Sherwill Sir Ambrose 75, 90
Slaughter houses 139
Smoking 17
Specialist Health Insurance Scheme 111, 121, 131
Speech Therapy Service 72
States
  Asylum Committee 59, 167
  Insurance Authority 122
  Supervisor 8, 37
St Johns Ambulance Association 48, 161
  Brigade 145, 146, 149
  first aiders 148
  personnel 98
St Johns Girls Industrial Home 51
St Peter Port Nursing Corps 49
Surgery 119
Symons Dr Angelo 54, 90, 101, 104, 109, 170

Thalasol 15
Thomas Dr A 17, 27, 75
Thompson Review 61
Tobacco control 18
Town Hospital - see Hospital
Tuberculosis 16, 69, 72, 84, 94, 101, 138
Typhoid 135
Typhus 135

'Undesirable aliens' 135
Uniforms 98, 149

Valnord
  House 46
  School 66, 77
Vauquiedor Estate 59, 167
Vauvert 63
Vega The 72
Venereal Diseases Clinic 94
Victoria Hotel Alderney 155

Water quality 11, 19
White Dr Geoffrey 16, 75
Wilson Mr Henry 105
Workhouse 31, 32, 91, 138, 157
World Health Organisation (WHO) 28

X-rays 120, 160, 171, 175